Safety and Microbiological Quality

Safety and Microbiological Quality

Special Issue Editors
Fabienne Remize
Didier Montet

MDPI • Basel • Beijing • Wuhan • Barcelona • Belgrade

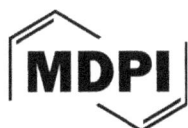

Special Issue Editors
Fabienne Remize
Université de La Réunion
France

Didier Montet
CIRAD
France

Editorial Office
MDPI
St. Alban-Anlage 66
4052 Basel, Switzerland

This is a reprint of articles from the Special Issue published online in the open access journal *Fermentation* (ISSN 2311-5637) from 2018 to 2019 (available at: https://www.mdpi.com/journal/fermentation/special_issues/safety_microbiological)

For citation purposes, cite each article independently as indicated on the article page online and as indicated below:

LastName, A.A.; LastName, B.B.; LastName, C.C. Article Title. *Journal Name* **Year**, *Article Number*, Page Range.

ISBN 978-3-03921-491-4 (Pbk)
ISBN 978-3-03921-492-1 (PDF)

Cover image courtesy of Fabienne Remiz.

© 2019 by the authors. Articles in this book are Open Access and distributed under the Creative Commons Attribution (CC BY) license, which allows users to download, copy and build upon published articles, as long as the author and publisher are properly credited, which ensures maximum dissemination and a wider impact of our publications.
The book as a whole is distributed by MDPI under the terms and conditions of the Creative Commons license CC BY-NC-ND.

Contents

About the Special Issue Editors vii

Fabienne Remize and Didier Montet
Safety and Microbiological Quality
Reprinted from: *fermentation* **2019**, *5*, 50, doi:10.3390/educsci5020050 1

Anil Kumar Anal
Quality Ingredients and Safety Concerns for Traditional Fermented Foods and Beverages from Asia: A Review
Reprinted from: *fermentation* **2019**, *5*, 8, doi:10.3390/educsci5010008 4

Pasquale Russo, Carmen Berbegal, Cristina De Ceglie, Francesco Grieco, Giuseppe Spano and Vittorio Capozzi
Pesticide Residues and Stuck Fermentation in Wine: New Evidences Indicate the Urgent Need of Tailored Regulations
Reprinted from: *fermentation* **2019**, *5*, 23, doi:10.3390/educsci5010023 16

Zuzana Matejčeková, Eva Vlková, Denisa Liptáková and Ľubomír Valík
Preliminary Screening of Growth and Viability of 10 Strains of *Bifidobacterium* spp.: Effect of Media Composition
Reprinted from: *fermentation* **2019**, *5*, 38, doi:10.3390/educsci5020038 28

Dimitrios A. Anagnostopoulos, Despina Bozoudi and Dimitrios Tsaltas
Enterococci Isolated from Cypriot Green Table Olives as a New Source of Technological and Probiotic Properties
Reprinted from: *fermentation* **2018**, *4*, 48, doi:10.3390/educsci4020048 39

Srijita Sireswar, Didier Montet and Gargi Dey
Principal Component Analysis for Clustering Probiotic-Fortified Beverage Matrices Efficient in Elimination of *Shigella* sp.
Reprinted from: *fermentation* **2018**, *5*, 34, doi:10.3390/educsci4020034 55

Alžbeta Medveďová, Petra Šipošová, Tatiana Mančušková and Ľubomír Valík
The Effect of Salt and Temperature on the Growth of Fresco Culture
Reprinted from: *fermentation* **2019**, *5*, 2, doi:10.3390/educsci5010002 64

Syed Ammar Hussain, Yusuf Nazir, Ahsan Hameed, Wu Yang, Kiren Mustafa and Yuanda Song
Optimization of Diverse Carbon Sources and Cultivation Conditions for Enhanced Growth and Lipid and Medium-Chain Fatty Acid (MCFA) Production by *Mucor circinelloides*
Reprinted from: *fermentation* **2019**, *5*, 35, doi:10.3390/educsci5020035 74

Elena Roselló-Soto, Cyrielle Garcia, Amandine Fessard, Francisco J. Barba, Paulo E. S. Munekata, Jose M. Lorenzo and Fabienne Remize
Nutritional and Microbiological Quality of Tiger Nut Tubers (*Cyperus esculentus*), Derived Plant-Based and Lactic Fermented Beverages
Reprinted from: *fermentation* **2019**, *5*, 3, doi:10.3390/educsci5010003 88

Jhoti Somanah, Manish Putteeraj, Okezie I. Aruoma and Theeshan Bahorun
Discovering the Health Promoting Potential of Fermented Papaya Preparation—Its Future Perspectives for the Dietary Management of Oxidative Stress During Diabetes
Reprinted from: *fermentation* **2018**, *4*, 83, doi:10.3390/educsci4040083 101

About the Special Issue Editors

Fabienne Remize studied food science and technology at the University of Montpellier (France). She earned her PhD in 1999, completed at INRA Montpellier on the regulation and engineering of glycerol production by *Saccharomyces cerevisiae* in wine. Following a post-doc at Gothenburg University (Sweden), she was appointed as an assistant professor at University of Burgundy (France), and focused her research activity on the adaptative metabolism of wine microorganisms and molecular tools applied to their detection. She worked for three years in the private sector and contributed to a better understanding of contamination pathways in canneries and the management of spoilage risk in canned foods. Since 2011, she has been a full professor at the University of La Réunion (France), studying microbial diversity in fruits and vegetables in order to preserve their quality and increase food shelf-life through environmentally friendly approaches.

Didier Montet earned his Ph.D. in food microbiology in 1984 at the University of Montpellier. Since then, he has been conducting research in the food industry and specifically in food safety for more than 35 years. He was the creator and team leader of Control of Contaminants along the Food Chain (Food Safety team) at CIRAD in Montpellier, France for 10 years. He is a national expert in biotechnology and additives at the National French Agency for Food Safety (Anses). He is the CIRAD representative for EFSA (article 36). His main research topic concerns the understanding of the microbial ecology of food and food safety. He has published nearly 160 papers and seven books as an editor in the field of food (fermentations, traceability). He has also run different European Projects (3C Ivoire) and participated in different European projects (Innovkar, After, Collab4safety, AsiFood, Autent-Net, Dafrali, Caravan). He was a food expert for the French Embassy in Southeast Asia and worked as a professor at the Asian Institute of Technology in Thailand (1997–1999). He has also worked with national food safety organizations around the world (including the FAO, French Embassy and several international NGO foundations). He developed a methodology of using collective expertise to identify food hazards that can be used, without high expenses, all over the world. This work has been published for Egypt, the Ivory Coast, Senegal, RD Congo, Morocco, and Southeast Asia. His work for the European Aid Project led to the creation of the Ivory Coast food agency in 2015. In 2018, he was enlisted by the French Embassy to help the government of the Philippines to build its food safety system of training. He was also enlisted by the FAO to help Mauritius to improve its food safety system.

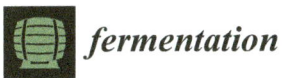

Editorial

Safety and Microbiological Quality

Fabienne Remize [1,*] and Didier Montet [2]

[1] UMR QualiSud, Université de La Réunion, CIRAD, Université Montpellier, Montpellier SupAgro, Université d'Avignon et des Pays de Vaucluse, 97490 Sainte Clotilde, France
[2] UMR QualiSud, CIRAD, Université Montpellier, Montpellier SupAgro, Université d'Avignon et des Pays de Vaucluse, Université de La Réunion, 34398 Montpellier CEDEX 5, France; didier.montet@cirad.fr
* Correspondence: fabienne.remize@univ-reunion.fr

Received: 12 June 2019; Accepted: 18 June 2019; Published: 19 June 2019

Food fermentation aims, primarily, to increase the shelf life of perishable foodstuffs. It is characterized by an extremely large diversity of raw materials, and an even wider range of fermented products, differing in their form, taste, color, or recipe [1]. The success of shelf life increase relies on acidification or ethanol production. Detoxification of endogenous compounds and increase in digestibility are other health-related benefits of fermentation. Additionally, in many parts of the word, as in Asia, fermented foods have a traditional role in overcoming food and nutritional insecurity [2].

Safety concerns cover the control of growth and persistence of foodborne pathogens, and the presence of toxic compounds, formed over fermentation or present in raw materials. For instance, in Italy, alcoholic fermentation during winemaking was affected by upstream plant treatments, i.e., pesticides used to fight *Plasmopara viticola*, the causal oomycete agent of grapevine downy mildew [3]. Active compounds used in commercial pesticide preparation, and possibly compounds used as excipients, negatively affect both *Saccharomyces* and non-*Saccharomyces* yeast growth. A careful examination of the effect on pro-technological microorganisms of pesticides is recommended.

Foodborne pathogen infections and diarrhea can be prevented with the use of probiotic cultures [4,5]. *Bifidobacterium* spp. is one of the most frequently used probiotic bacteria. Probiotic effect requires that the bacteria can survive and grow in the food matrix used for probiotic delivery. Hence, examination of *Bifidobacterium* strain viability in media is a key component for probiotic development [6]. Similarly, *Enterococcus faecium* and *Enterococcus faecalis* are frequently isolated from fermented foods, for instance table olives [7]. In addition, they produce bile salt hydrolases and are resistant to low pH, and are therefore able to stay alive until they reach the intestinal tract. However, these two Gram-positive lactic acid bacteria have been implicated in infectious diseases and a careful examination of antibiotic susceptibility, virulence, and absence of hemolysis and cytotoxicity is required before their use as starters and possibly probiotics [8–10].

The use of fruit juice to deliver probiotics is an advantage regarding lactose intolerant people and, for economic reasons, in developing countries. An innovative strategy for the prevention of shigellosis, which persists endemically and causes epidemics in tropical countries, is to enhance the capacity of probiotics to suppress the growth of different species of *Shigella*. This approach was applied with different fruit matrix, and the impact of processing and the storage of the juice on the efficacy of probiotics was examined [11].

Microbiological quality of fermented foods includes fermentation process reliability, which impacts sensory quality and shelf life. Process reliability depends on starter fitness and its growth properties in the food matrix. Predictive growth models can be used to determine the optimal conditions on use of single or mixed lactic acid bacterium cultures [12]. In addition, microbiological quality of fermented foods and beverages is closely connected to nutritional quality. For instance, the fungus *Mucor circinelloides* is a promising oil cell factory, producing medium-chain fatty acids (MCFA). Adjustment of cultivation conditions can improve biomass, total fatty acid, and MCFA contents [13].

The development of new lactic fermented beverages from non-dairy sources is of increasing interest because of the combined advantages of plant nutritional properties and benefits from lactic fermentation [14,15]. Tiger nut tubers, *Cyperus esculentus*, are of particular interest because of their richness in lipid and dietary fiber, close to those of nuts, a high content of starch, like in other tubers, and high levels of phosphorus, calcium, and phenolic compounds [16]. The development of fermented or probiotic beverages from tiger nuts must carefully select a tailored bacterial cocktail able to dominate undesirable endogenous flora (either foodborne pathogens or spoilage microorganisms), preserve bioactive compounds, and result in a well-accepted beverage. The nutritional properties of fermented papaya have been extensively studied over the last decade. At present, a corpus of studies shows the cellular protective effects of fermented papaya and its ability to reduce oxidative stress, and thinking of the use of that product for disease prevention and management through a holistic approach has been reviewed [17,18].

All together, the articles of this special issue provide a broad view of the safety and microbiological quality determining factors in fermented foods. The interconnection of starter properties and probiotic effect expectations are focused on. A common point of the articles published in this special issue is their involvement towards better resource management and increasing food and nutritional security, especially in developing countries.

Conflicts of Interest: The authors declare no conflict of interest.

References

1. Ray, R.C.; Montet, D. *Microorganisms and Fermentation of Traditional Foods*; CRC Press: Boca Raton, FL, USA, 2015; ISBN 9781482223088.
2. Kumar Anal, A. Quality Ingredients and Safety Concerns for Traditional Fermented Foods and Beverages from Asia: A Review. *Fermentation* **2019**, *5*, 8. [CrossRef]
3. Russo, P.; Berbegal, C.; De Ceglie, C.; Grieco, F.; Spano, G.; Capozzi, V.; Russo, P.; Berbegal, C.; De Ceglie, C.; Grieco, F.; et al. Pesticide Residues and Stuck Fermentation in Wine: New Evidences Indicate the Urgent Need of Tailored Regulations. *Fermentation* **2019**, *5*, 23. [CrossRef]
4. Ranadheera, C.; Vidanarachchi, J.; Rocha, R.; Cruz, A.; Ajlouni, S.; Ranadheera, C.S.; Vidanarachchi, J.K.; Rocha, R.S.; Cruz, A.G.; Ajlouni, S. Probiotic Delivery through Fermentation: Dairy vs. Non-Dairy Beverages. *Fermentation* **2017**, *3*, 67. [CrossRef]
5. Hill, C.; Guarner, F.; Reid, G.; Gibson, G.R.; Merenstein, D.J.; Pot, B.; Morelli, L.; Canani, R.B.; Flint, H.J.; Salminen, S.; et al. The International Scientific Association for Probiotics and Prebiotics consensus statement on the scope and appropriate use of the term probiotic. *Nat. Rev. Gastroenterol. Hepatol.* **2014**, *11*, 506–514. [CrossRef] [PubMed]
6. Matejčeková, Z.; Vlková, E.; Liptáková, D.; Valík, Ľ. Preliminary Screening of Growth and Viability of 10 Strains of *Bifidobacterium* sp.: Effect of Media Composition. *Fermentation* **2019**, *5*, 38. [CrossRef]
7. Anagnostopoulos, D.; Bozoudi, D.; Tsaltas, D.; Anagnostopoulos, D.A.; Bozoudi, D.; Tsaltas, D. Enterococci Isolated from Cypriot Green Table Olives as a New Source of Technological and Probiotic Properties. *Fermentation* **2018**, *4*, 48. [CrossRef]
8. Foulquié Moreno, M.R.; Sarantinopoulos, P.; Tsakalidou, E.; De Vuyst, L. The role and application of enterococci in food and health. *Int. J. Food Microbiol.* **2006**, *106*, 1–24. [CrossRef] [PubMed]
9. Baccouri, O.; Boukerb, A.M.; Farhat, L.B.; Zébré, A.; Zimmermann, K.; Domann, E.; Cambronel, M.; Barreau, M.; Maillot, O.; Rincé, I.; et al. Probiotic Potential and Safety Evaluation of *Enterococcus faecalis* OB14 and OB15, Isolated from Traditional Tunisian Testouri Cheese and Rigouta, Using Physiological and Genomic Analysis. *Front. Microbiol.* **2019**, *10*, 881. [CrossRef] [PubMed]
10. Ayala, D.I.; Cook, P.W.; Franco, J.G.; Bugarel, M.; Kottapalli, K.R.; Loneragan, G.H.; Brashears, M.M.; Nightingale, K.K. A Systematic Approach to Identify and Characterize the Effectiveness and Safety of Novel Probiotic Strains to Control Foodborne Pathogens. *Front. Microbiol.* **2019**, *10*, 1108. [CrossRef] [PubMed]
11. Sireswar, S.; Montet, D.; Dey, G.; Sireswar, S.; Montet, D.; Dey, G. Principal Component Analysis for Clustering Probiotic-Fortified Beverage Matrices Efficient in Elimination of *Shigella* sp. *Fermentation* **2018**, *4*, 34. [CrossRef]

12. Medveďová, A.; Šipošová, P.; Mančušková, T.; Valík, Ľ. The Effect of Salt and Temperature on the Growth of Fresco Culture. *Fermentation* **2018**, *5*, 2. [CrossRef]
13. Hussain, S.A.; Nazir, Y.; Hameed, A.; Yang, W.; Mustafa, K.; Song, Y.; Hussain, S.A.; Nazir, Y.; Hameed, A.; Yang, W.; et al. Optimization of Diverse Carbon Sources and Cultivation Conditions for Enhanced Growth and Lipid and Medium-Chain Fatty Acid (MCFA) Production by *Mucor circinelloides*. *Fermentation* **2019**, *5*, 35. [CrossRef]
14. Fessard, A.; Kapoor, A.; Patche, J.; Assemat, S.; Hoarau, M.; Bourdon, E.; Bahorun, T.; Remize, F. Lactic fermentation as an efficient tool to enhance the antioxidant activity of tropical fruit juices and teas. *Microorganisms* **2017**, *5*, 23. [CrossRef] [PubMed]
15. Septembre-Malaterre, A.; Remize, F.; Poucheret, P. Fruits and vegetables, as a source of nutritional compounds and phytochemicals: Changes in bioactive compounds during lactic fermentation. *Food Res. Int.* **2017**. [CrossRef] [PubMed]
16. Roselló-Soto, E.; Garcia, C.; Fessard, A.; Barba, F.; Munekata, P.; Lorenzo, J.; Remize, F.; Roselló-Soto, E.; Garcia, C.; Fessard, A.; et al. Nutritional and Microbiological Quality of Tiger Nut Tubers (*Cyperus esculentus*), Derived Plant-Based and Lactic Fermented Beverages. *Fermentation* **2019**, *5*, 3. [CrossRef]
17. Somanah, J.; Putteeraj, M.; Aruoma, O.; Bahorun, T.; Somanah, J.; Putteeraj, M.; Aruoma, O.I.; Bahorun, T. Discovering the Health Promoting Potential of Fermented Papaya Preparation—Its Future Perspectives for the Dietary Management of Oxidative Stress During Diabetes. *Fermentation* **2018**, *4*, 83. [CrossRef]
18. Somanah, J.; Bourdon, E.; Rondeau, P.; Bahorun, T.; Aruoma, O.I. Relationship between fermented papaya preparation supplementation, erythrocyte integrity and antioxidant status in pre-diabetics. *Food Chem. Toxicol.* **2014**, *65*, 12–17. [CrossRef] [PubMed]

© 2019 by the authors. Licensee MDPI, Basel, Switzerland. This article is an open access article distributed under the terms and conditions of the Creative Commons Attribution (CC BY) license (http://creativecommons.org/licenses/by/4.0/).

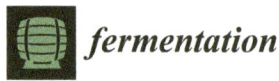

Review

Quality Ingredients and Safety Concerns for Traditional Fermented Foods and Beverages from Asia: A Review

Anil Kumar Anal

Food Engineering and Bioprocess Technology, Department of Food, Agriculture and Bioresources, Asian Institute of Technology, PO Box 4, Klong Luang, Pathumthani 12120, Thailand; anilkumar@ait.ac.th

Received: 22 November 2018; Accepted: 2 January 2019; Published: 10 January 2019

Abstract: Fermented foods and beverages serve as vehicles for beneficial microorganisms that play an important role in human health and remain the oldest prevalent means of food processing and preservation. Traditional fermented foods are popular in Asia for their nutritional balance and food security. Techniques for preserving cereals, vegetables, and meat products are well developed in many Asian countries. Due to their cultural and nutritional significance, many of these foods have been studied in detail and their quality and safety have also been improved. These fermented foods and beverages provide benefits through enhanced nutritional content, digestibility, microbial stability, and detoxification. They represent is thus one of the most affordable and suitable methods to maintain hygiene condition and food quality and security in poor and underdeveloped countries. There is an industrial interest and scope related to traditional fermented foods and beverages in Asia. However, urgent attention is required to improve the quality of the ingredients and the integration of food safety management systems for industrial growth.

Keywords: fermentation; traditional; nutritional value; microbiology; Asian countries

1. Introduction

Indigenous fermented foods and beverages have been part of the human diet since the beginning of civilization. Such foods are either served as staples or adjuncts to staples, pickles, condiments, and beverages. Fermentation dates back to the Neolithic period (circa 10,000 B.C.), when it was used primarily for the preservation of perishable food. Microorganisms were generally inoculated to use for the fermentation and maturation of foods. Fermentation was primarily aimed for food preservation, obtained by the formation of inhibitory metabolites, such as organic acid, ethanol, and bacteriocins, in combination with reduced water activity. However, fermentation has been explored for other functions such as improvement in food safety through the inhibition of pathogens or removal of toxic compounds; improvement in nutritional value; and improvement in the organoleptic quality of the food [1]. In addition, fermentation provides a natural way to reduce the volume of the material to be transported, to destroy undesirable components, to enhance the nutritive value and appearance of the food, to reduce the energy required for cooking, and to make a safer product.

Fermented food products are produced widely using different techniques, raw materials, and microorganisms. However, there are basically only four types of fermentation processes involved in the product development, namely, alcoholic, lactic acid, acetic acid, and alkali fermentation, as described below.

Lactic acid fermentation is mainly carried out by lactic acid bacteria (LAB). Examples include fermented cereals, *kimchi*, sauerkraut, and *gundruk*.

Alcohol fermentation contributes to the production of ethanol. Yeasts are the predominant organisms, for example, wines, beers, vodka, whiskey, brandy, and bread.

Acetic acid fermentation is produced from the *Acetobacter* species. *Acetobacter* converts alcohol to acetic acid in the presence of oxygen (e.g., vinegar).

Alkaline fermentation takes place during the fermentation of soybeans, fish, and seeds, popularly used as a condiment.

Fermented foods are associated with a unique group of microflora that enhance the nutritional quality of food such as proteins, vitamins, essential amino acids, and fatty acids. On the other hand, three quarters of humanity are deprived of basic food and are malnourished. In this regard, fermented food products can address the problems related to the world's balanced diet [2]. Fermented food products are typically unique and vary depending on the region due to the variation in environmental conditions, cultural and social aspects, taste preferences, availability of raw materials, and new technological development [3]. Based on raw materials available, different types of fermented food products are prepared to increase food varieties in order to overcome food and nutrition insecurity.

Asia is well known for its techniques to preserve and balance the fluctuation in food availability during the monsoonal circulation. Paddy production in Southeast Asian countries accounts for 25% of world production (150 million tons per year) of which 95% is consumed within the region. The fermentation of cereals and other plant products to produce a variety of foods is a common practice since ancient times. Rice wine is one of the popular fermented beverages and fermented cassava tubers is another of the many fermented food products widely consumed in Asian countries [4].

Fermented foods and beverages may vary based on the nature of the food, the fermentation time, and the intentional application of microbes utilized. Fermentation could occur at the starting process for products that undergo multiple additional steps once the fermentation is terminated, such as in coffee, chocolate, tea leaves, sourdough bread products, among others (Table 1). On the other hand, fermentation could continue to characterize the final products, such as in pungent-smelling blue cheese or vinegar-tasting kombucha [5].

Table 1. Examples of common fermented foods and beverages developed during process and/or as final products.

Fermentation in the Preparation Phase	Fermentation of the Final Food Product
Coffee	Soy Sauce
Chocolate	Yogurt
Fermented tea leaves	Kimchi
Sourdough bread	Kombucha, beer, wine

Fermentation is utilized in the preparation phase typically in products such as chocolate and coffee. Chocolate is made from the fermentation of cocoa beans with the successive action of yeast, acetic acid bacteria (AAB), and lactic acid bacteria (LAB) driving the conversion of pulp substrate into ethanol, lactic acid, and acetic acid. During fermentation, flavor and aroma precursors develop and pigments are degraded by the action of enzymes such as invertases, glycosidases, proteases, and polyphenol oxidase. Fermentation influences the compounds such as reducing sugars, peptides, and amino acids, which are converted into flavor and smell profiles during the drying and roasting steps of chocolate processing [6]. Tea is a rich source of several flavonoid compounds that are responsible for its distinctive taste and color along with various health benefits. In a research study by Jayasekera et al. [7], total catechins, total flavonols, and total theaflavins were observed to be higher in fermented Sri Lankan tea leaves compared to the unfermented tea leaves. Traditionally, coffee beans are fermented to remove mucilage and prepare the beans for roasting. However, the fermentation also helps in the development of the coffee's aroma quality.

Figure 1 illustrates the schematic representation of types of fermentation, the microorganisms involved, and the resulting end products. Based on raw materials, manufacturing techniques, and microorganisms, various types of fermented food products are available. During alcoholic fermentation, yeasts are the predominant microorganisms and result in the production of ethanol.

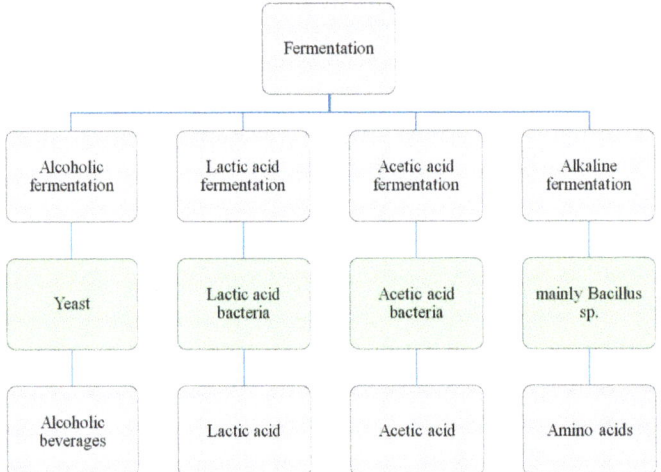

Figure 1. Schematic representation of the common types of fermentation, the microorganisms involved, and the end products.

Lactic acid fermentation is mainly carried out by lactic acid bacteria (LAB). The acetic acid fermentation by acetic acid producers from the *Acetobacter* species converts alcohol to acetic acid in the presence of excess oxygen. Alkali fermentation often takes place during the fermentation of fish and seeds, popularly used as condiments [8].

2. Quality Attributes of Common Fermented Foods of Asia

The prevalence of malnutrition and nutritional deficiencies are common problems in developing and underdeveloped countries. The lack of proper dietary quality, an inadequate food consumption, a lower nutrient bioavailability, and the outbreak of infectious diseases are considered to be the major reasons for malnutrition. Furthermore, concerns about food safety regarding microbial contamination and naturally occurring toxins are of great importance. To combat these problems, simple, cost-effective, and indigenous food-based approaches such as the fermentation process are considered to be effective. The fermentation process improves the nutritional quality, digestibility, and bioavailability of nutrients, while also reducing anti-nutritional factors and enhancing the shelf life and safety of the product [9].

2.1. Alcoholic Fermented Foods and Beverages

Alcoholic fermentation has been practiced since ancient times and is therefore one of the oldest and most important techniques in food processing. This process results in the production of various alcoholic beverages like beers, wines, and distilled liquors, using yeast or sometimes yeast-like molds, such as *Amylomyces rouxii*, and mold-like yeasts such as *Endomycopsis* and bacteria such as *Zymomonas mobilis*. These microorganisms involve the utilization of fermentable sugars from substrates such as cereal grains, sugar cane juice, palm sap, fruit juices, diluted honey, or hydrolyzed starch, resulting in the production of mainly ethanol and carbon dioxide.

In Asia, there are at least two additional ways of fermenting starch rice to obtain alcohol: first, the starch is converted to simple sugars by the action of amylase enzymes produced by mold such as *Amylomyces rouxii*, followed by the fermentation of sugars to ethanol by the action of yeast such as *Endomycopsis fibuliger*. Rice, inflorescences of palm such as coconut and *talipot* palm, millet, and others are common substrates for the production of alcoholic beverages.

The wines from coconut and *talipot* palm are commonly produced all over Asia. The fermented beverage from palm saps is called *"panam culloo"* in Vietnam, *"arak"* in Indonesia, and *"tuak"* or toddy in Malaysia, India, and Bangladesh. Toddy is the traditional fermented alcoholic beverage made by fermenting the sap from the coconut, palmyra, and toddy palm. The tip of an unopened flower is sliced, causing sap to ooze out from the cut and which is then collected in an earthenware container tied underneath the flower. The sap can be consumed either as fresh sap or allowed to ferment for up to 24 h. The fresh sap is a dirty-brown sweet liquid with a sugar content of approximately 10%–18% w/w which on formation results in an alcoholic beverage with an ethanol content of as much as 9% (v/v) [10]. Palm wine is one of the cheapest sources of vitamin B for the poorer communities; it contains 0.019%–0.028% (w/v) of vitamin B-12 and 0.008% of ascorbic acid. The amounts of thiamine, riboflavin, and pyridoxine increase with fermentation [4]. Fermented coconut toddy contains approximately 1.8–7.9 g alcohol, 0.29 g sucrose, 0.9–3.0 g invert sugar, and 3.72 g/dL total solids. It contains nitrogen, phosphorus, potassium, calcium, and magnesium <0.5 g/100 mL [11]. The palm sap fermentation process involves alcoholic-lactic-acetic acid fermentation in the presence of mainly yeasts and LAB. The yeast species *Saccharomyces cerevisiae* is invariably present along with other LAB such as *Lactobacillus plantarum*, *Lactobacillus mesenteroides*, or other species of bacteria such as *Zymomonas mobilis* and *Acetobacter* spp. [10]. In coconut sap fermentation, *Saccharomyces chevalieri* is the main alcohol producer [11]. The common traditionally fermented alcoholic beverages in Asia are summarized in Table 2.

Table 2. Common fermented alcoholic beverages in Asia.

Country	Raw Materials	Local Name	Microorganism	References
Bangladesh	Rice Palm	Bangla maad Tari	Yeast *S. cerevisiae*; *L. plantarum*, *L. mesenteroides*; *Zymomonas mobilis*, *Acetobacter* spp.	[10]
Sri Lanka	Coconut, palmyra, or *Caryota urens* flower sap	Toddy	*S. exiguus*, *S. cerevisiae*, *Pichia fermentans*, *S. rosei*, *S. fructuum*, *Torulopsis holmii*, *Torulopsis versatilis*, *Candida robusta*, *Candida lambica*, *Saccharomyces*, *Schizosaccharomyces*, *Brettanomyces*	[11]
Nepal	Millet, rice, buckwheat	Jaand	*Aspergillus oryzae*, LAB, ethanol-fermenting yeast	[12]
	Millet, rice, buckwheat	Rakshi	Saccharifying molds, LAB, ethanol fermenting yeast	
	Rice	Hyaun thon	*Aspergillus oryzae*, *Rhizopus* spp., LAB	
Thailand	Glutinous rice, Loogpaeng	Sato (rice wine)	*Amylomyces* sp., *Aspergillus* sp., *Rhizopus* sp., *S. cerevisiae*	[13]
Japan	Rice	Sake	*A. oryzae*, *S. cerevisiae*, *L. plantarum*, *L. leichmanii*	[14]
Vietnam	Rice Glutinous rice	Ruou de Ruou nep	*Mucor* spp., *Rhizopus* spp., *Aspergillus* spp., *S. ellipsoideus*, *S. cerevisiae*, *Endomycopsis fibuliger*, *Hansenula anomala*, *Torulopsis candida*	[15]

Some of the traditional alcoholic beverages of Nepal include *Jaand*, *Rakshi*, and *Huaun thon*. *Jaand* or *jaanr* is an undistilled alcoholic beverage made from different raw materials such as rice, millet, maize, wheat, and other starch-rich substrates by the action of a starter known as *murcha*. The distilled alcoholic beverage with a characteristic aroma from *jaand* is known as *rakshi*. The major microorganisms present in *murcha* are filamentous molds such as *Mucor circinelloides*, *M. hiemalis*, *Rhizopus chinensis*, and *R. stolonifer* var. *lyococcus*; yeasts such as *S. fibuligera*, *S. capsularis*, *Pichia anomala*, *P. burtonii*, *S. cerevisiae*,

S. bayanus, and *C. glabrata*; and LAB such as *P. pentosaceus*, *Lactobacillus bifermentans*, and *L. brevi*. *Jaand* contains 5%–9% alcohol, 0.8%–1.1% acidity (as lactic acid), 1.6%–2.5% reducing sugar as glucose, 1.6%–2.8% total sugar (as sucrose), 12%–14% starch, and 76%–80% water. In the final fermented product, protein content increased up to 17.6%–38.8%; carbohydrate content decreased 86.41% to about 77.29%–77.71%; thiamine content increased up to 16%–32%; pyridoxine content increased by 50%–59%; niacin content increased up to 117%–173%; and the increase in folic acid was nearly 76% [12].

In Thailand, rice is the main crop and is harvested one or two times per year. *Sato* is the traditional alcoholic beverage of Thailand prepared from glutinous rice, a starter culture (*Loogpaeng*), and water. *Loogpaeng* as the starter culture contains different kinds of microorganisms such as fungi, yeast, and bacteria. Dominant fungi are *Aspergillus*, *Mucor*, *Rhizopus*, *Amylomyces*, and *Penicillium*, while *Endomycopsis* and *Saccharomyces* are the existing yeasts in *Loogpaeng*. Along with these, acetic acid bacteria (AAB), LAB and *Bacillus* are also detected in the starter culture. During *sato* production, once the cooked glutinous rice is mixed with *Loogpaeng*, it starts to become turbid and sweet due to the saccharification caused by the amylase enzyme produced by *Amylomyces* and *Rhizopus*. After the addition of water to the sweet rice, yeast including bacteria starts to grow leading to alcoholic fermentation. Depending on the quality of *Loogpaeng*, alcohol content is about 7%–10% (v/v) in the final fermented product [13]. *Khoaw Maak* is another popular traditionally fermented Thai dessert made from fermented rice. It is acidic sweet in taste and white in appearance. A research study was conducted to evaluate the bioactive components of the Thai rice fermentation. *Oryza sativa* L. var. *indica*, including white plain, purple plain, brown plain, white glutinous, and purple glutinous rice, was fermented with Look-Pang (a mixed culture of yeasts and molds). The sap sample from the fermentation of the purple plain rice showed the highest free radical scavenging (the sample concentrations that scavenged 50% of the DPPH radicals, SC_{50} at 14.51 ± 2.21 mg/mL), as well as tyrosinase inhibition (the sample concentrations that inhibited 50% of tyrosinase activity, IC_{50} at 15.05 ± 2.92 mg/mL) and MMP-2 inhibition activities (62.22% ± 3.78%). Tyrosinase is the main enzyme that catalyzes the melanin synthesis. Matrix metalloproteinases (MMPs) are enzymes which degrade the collagen matrix, in addition to reducing arthritis, inflammation, heart-related diseases, cancer, and skin aging. Many MMP inhibitors are basically vitamin C and vitamin E [16].

Similar traditional rice wines have equivalent appellations, such as Japanese *Sake* and *Mirin*, Vietnamese *Ruou*, Philippine *Tapuy*, Indonesian *Brem*, Malaysian *Tapai*, Korean *Makkulli* and *Yakju*, and Chinese *Huang jiu*, *Huadiao jiu*, *Shaohsing*, *Chia Fan*, *Hsiang Hsueh*, *Shan Niang*, and *Yen Hung* [17]. *Sake* is the traditional alcoholic rice beverage prepared and consumed in Japan and China. The seed mash for *Sake* preparation is traditionally obtained by natural lactic acid fermentation involving various aerobic bacteria, wild yeasts, LAB, and sake yeast [8]. During *Sake* brewing, saccharification and alcoholic fermentation progress simultaneously. The starter, *koji*, is rich in enzyme activity including amylases and proteases. From a nutritional point of view, *Sake* is distinctive among alcoholic beverages as it contains more proteins (0.4 g/100 g) and carbohydrates (4.1 g/100 g) that make it richer in taste than other beverages [14]. The rice wines *ruou de* or *ruou nep*, fermented from rice or glutinous rice, are popular traditional alcoholic beverages in Vietnam. The starters used for fermenting *ruou de* or *ruou nep* include yeasts, molds, and bacteria that convert starch material to fermentable sugars, which are subsequently converted to alcohol and organic acids. The alcohol content of these traditional undistilled wines is around 7%–10% (v/v) [15].

Herbs are known as rich sources of bioactive compounds entering in the preparation of traditional beverages (antioxidant, anti-inflammatory, antimicrobial). Traditional date juice (*Phoenix dactylifera*), Tassabount in Morocco, is a preparation using medicinal and aromatic plant macerate which is fermented for 3–5 days. A variety of plants are used including more than 20 species (basil, clove, thyme, lemon, iris, mythe, oregano, nutmeg, rosemary, mandrak). The fermentation process has the potential to produce new beneficial compounds, resulting in the increase of biological properties of traditional preparations. This aromatic extract has been reported to contain bioactive compounds such as carvacrol, thymol, and phenolic compounds providing antimicrobial properties and improving the safety status and shelf life of the traditional juice [18,19].

Angkak or red yeast rice has been used extensively in Asian cuisine as a natural food colorant in fish, Chinese cheese, red wine, and sausages. *Angkak* is a product of the solid-state fermentation of rice by *Monasus* fungi which can convert starchy substrates into metabolites such as alcohols, antibiotic agents, antihypertensives, enzymes, fatty acids, flavor compounds, organic acids, pigments, and vitamins. *Angkak* contains mevinolin, a compound that inhibits cholesterol production by blocking a key enzyme, HMG-Coa reductase. However, another secondary metabolite, known as citrinin ($C_{13}H_{14}O_5$) which is a hepato-nephrotoxin, is also synthesized by *Monascus* strains [20]. The new product from an adlay substrate (Chinese pearl barley) fermented by *Monascus purpureus* produced the adlay angkak with the lowest citrinin and the highest mevinolin content [21]. The study showed the positive effect of the fermented papaya preparation (FPP) on Type 2 diabetes [22]. FPP was made from the yeast fermentation of ripen papaya using a specialized biotechnological technique. The evaluation was conducted by studying its effect on the human antioxidant status and erythrocyte integrity of a multi-ethnical pre-diabetic population. Fermented papaya exhibited effective in vitro free radical scavenging activities, believed to be attributed to the residual phenolic or flavonoid compounds.

2.2. Lactic Acid Fermentation

Lactic acid bacteria (LAB) belong to a group of Gram-positive facultative anaerobic bacteria that synthesize lactic acid as their main product of fermentation into the culture medium. Lactic acid fermentation is performed by LAB of which the genera are mostly composed of *Lactobacillus*, *Lactococcus*, *Enterococcus*, *Streptococcus*, *Pediococcus*, *Leuconostoc*, *Weisiella*, etc. Lactic acid bacteria assist in preserving and producing a wide range of foods. Traditional uses of many LAB as fermentation agents for foods are considered to be safe for the general population. Lactic acid bacteria cause rapid acidification of food due to the production of acids, primarily lactic acid. Other metabolites associated with LAB include acetic acid, ethanol, aromatic compounds, bacteriocins, exopolysaccharides, and several enzymes. These compounds result in the enhancement of shelf life and microbial safety, as well as the improvement of texture and sensory profile of the fermented products. Different fermented products are available that come mainly from lactic acid fermentation: fermented dairy products (cheese, butter, and butter milk, yoghurt, fermented probiotic milk, kefir); fermented meat products (sausages); fermented fish products; fermented fresh vegetables such as cabbage (sauerkraut, *kimchi*); cucumbers (pickles); fermented cereals (sourdough bread and bread-like products); and alcoholic beverages (wine) [23]. Moreover, because of their ability to produce lactic acid, up to 50 different species of *Lactobacillus plantarum* have been applied to popular traditional fermentation food technology for products such as meat, vegetables and dairy. Furthermore, improving the conversion, flavor and texture characteristics of fermented food are considered as main reasons for using this probiotic strain in industrial food technology. Tailor-made LABs with desired physiological traits can be constructed and applied to optimize the food manufacturing processes or to manipulate the organoleptic properties (i.e., the overall flavor and texture) of the products. Table 3 summarizes the common lactic acid-fermented food products in Asia.

Kefir is a traditional milk product, the combination of lactic acid bacteria and yeast. Special taste and aroma were found in a kefir product, the combination of lactic acid and alcohol. In addition, fresh milk was usually fermented by the kefir grain, insoluble in water and containing a group of microorganisms. Moreover, *Lactobacillus* species are considered as the majority of bacteria in kefir. Therefore, the kefir product was recognized as containing antimicrobial activity because kefir grain produces antibacterial metabolites such as lactic acid, volatile acids, hydrogen peroxide, carbon dioxide, diacetyl, and acetaldehyde. Many studies have focused on research into the survival capacity of LAB in cereal and fruit materials such as oat flour, malt, barley, and cabbage juice. The fruits and vegetables are considered as rich functional components such as minerals, vitamins, dietary fiber, and antioxidants. It is recognized that lactic acid milk fermentation can generate a large number of peptides with potentially bioactive properties. Quirós et al. [26] fermented milk with different strains of *E. faecalis* and identified two peptides, corresponding to β-casein f(133–138) and β-casein f(58–76). These peptides demonstrated angiotensin converting enzyme-inhibitory (ACEI) activity. Furthermore, when administered orally to hypertensive rats, the peptides exhibited antihypertensive activity.

Table 3. Common lactic acid-fermented food products in Asia.

Country	Raw Materials	Local Name	Microorganism	References
Cereal Grains				
Nepal	Rice	Selroti	Lactobacillus curvatus, Pseudomonas pentosaceuts, Escherecia faecium, Saccharomyces cerevisiae, Saccharomyces kluyveri, Debaryomyces hansenii, Pichia burtonii, Zygosaccharomyces rouxii	[24]
India	Rice Black gram	Idli Dosa	Leuconostoc mesenteroides, Streptococcus faecali, Pediococcus cerevisiae	
Vegetables				
Nepal	Cabbage, cauliflower, radish, mustard leaf	Gundruk	Pediococcus pentasaceous, Lactobacillus cellubiosus, and Lactobacillus plantarum	
Korea	Cabbage, radish, various vegetables	Kimchi	Leuconostoc mesenteroides, Lactobacillus brevis, Lactobacillus plantarum	
Vietnam	Cabbage	Dhamuoi	Leuconostoc. mesenteroides, Lactobacillus plantarum	
Thailand	Mustard leaf	Dakguadong	Lactobacillus plantarum	
Philippines	Mustard leaf	Burong mustala	Lactobacillus brevis, Pediococcus cerevisiae	
Meat and Fish Products				
Philippines	Fresh water fish, rice,	Burong-isda	Lactobacillus brevis Streptococcus sp.	
Thailand	Fresh water fish, salt, steamed rice	Som-fak Pla-ra	Pediococcus sp. and Lactobacillus sp.	
	Shrimp, salt, sweetened rice	Kungchao	Pediococcus cerevisiae	
	Pork, garlic, salt, rice	Nham	Pediococcus cerevisiae Lactobacillus plantarum Lactobacillus brevis	[25]
Korea	Sea water fish, cooked millet, salt	Sikhae	Leuconostoc mesenteroides Lactobacillus plantarum	
Japan	Sea water fish, cooked millet, salt	Narezushi	Leuconostoc mesenteroides Lactobacillus plantarum	
Vietnam	Pork, salt, cooked rice	Nem-chua	Pediococcus sp. Lactobacillus sp.	

Cereal products can be fermented either to produce alcoholic beverages or non-alcoholic food products mostly in the form of breads, loaves, confectionery, and gruels, or as complementary foods for infants and children. Non-alcoholic fermented cereal products include sourdough of America,

Europe, Australia; *dosa* and *idli* of India; *puto* of Southeast Asia; *masa* of South Africa; *kisra* of Sudan; *tarhana* of Turkey, and so on. Among the Nepalese people, fermented cereal food called *selroti*, which is prepared from rice, is quite popular. Yonzan and Tamang [24] studied the microbiology and nutritional values of *selroti* with the long-term goal of developing a good starter culture technology. The LAB strain, comprising lactobacilli, pediococci, leuconostocs, and enterococci, and the yeast strains *S. cerevisiae, S. kluyveri, D. hansenii, P. burtonii*, and *Z. rouxii* were found to co-exist as the predominant microorganisms. With fermentation, water-soluble and tricholoroacetic acid (TCA) soluble nitrogen were observed to increase, indicating an enhancement in protein digestibility.

Fermentation enhances the functional properties as well as the food value of the product. Indian *idli* and *dosa* are the traditional products made from polished rice and dehulled black gram by lactic acid fermentation. Both are products of natural lactic acid fermentation by *L. mesenteroides* and *S. faecalis*. Within the fermentation time of 20 h, the reduction of sugars (such as glucose) was observed, decreasing from 3.3 mg/g of dry ingredients to 0.8 mg/g, reflecting the utilization of sugar for acid and gas production. Flatulence-causing oligosaccharides, such as stachyose and raffinose, were found completely hydrolyzed. A decrease in phytate phosphorous and an increase in thiamine and riboflavin have also been reported during fermentation in the same study.

Gundruk is a non-salted fermented and dried vegetable product of Nepal. It is prepared by spontaneous lactic acid fermentation of green leafy vegetables, including the leaves of *Brassica* species such as mustard (*Brassica campestris* L.), rayo (*B. juncea* L.), cauliflower (*B. campestris* L. var. *botrytis* L.), cabbage (*B. oleracea* L, and radish (*Raphanus sativus* L.) [27]. *Gundruk* is one of the highly priced indigenous products of Nepal. It is served as a side dish with the main meal, as an appetizer, and as a soup. The annual production of *Gundruk* in Nepal is estimated at 2000 tons and most of the production is carried out at the household level. *Pediococcus pentasaceous, Lactobacillus cellubiosus*, and *Lactobacillus plantarum* are the dominant microorganisms in *Gundruk* fermentation. The pH values of *Gundruk* prepared from mustard, rape, and radish leaves were 4.0, 4.3, and 4.1, respectively, and the lactic acid contents were 1.0, 0.8, and 0.9%, respectively [12].

Traditionally fermented lightly salted fish products composed of fish, salt (2%–7%), carbohydrate source (rice, millet, sugar), and spices (garlic, ginger, chili, pepper) are popular in Southeast Asia. *Som-fak* is a traditional Thai product composed of fish fillet, salt (2%–5%), ground boiled rice (2%–12%), and minced garlic (4%). The mixtures are tightly packed in banana leaves and allowed to ferment at ambient temperature for 2–4 days. Rapid growth of LAB drops pH below 4.5, and *Pediococcus sp.* and *Lactobacillus* sp. have been identified as the dominating LAB [28]. Ribas-Agustí et al. [29] developed fermented sausage with the addition of vegetable extract, cocoa extract, and grape seed extract (GSE) with the aim of producing fermented meat with a balanced quantity of phenolic and other bio-active compounds. After completing the aging process, catechin and epicatechin were at 54%–61%, gallic acid and galloylated flavan-3-ols were at 59%–91%, oligomeric flavan-3-ols were at 72%–95%, and glycosylated flavonols were at 56%–88% (in cocoa treatment), as well as 82%–94% (in GSE treatment) of the contents that were added to the meat batter.

2.3. Acetic Acid Fermentation

Acetic acid bacteria (AAB) are also commonly found in a wide range of fermented foods and beverages. AAB are ubiquitous, aerobic, Gram-negative bacteria belonging to the *Acetobacteraceae*, and the genera *Acetobacter, Gluconobacter, Gluconacetobacter*, and *Komagataeibacter* constitute the common AAB found in food and beverage fermentation such as cocoa, milk kefir, water kefir, kombucha, and acidic beers [30]. AAB are predominantly known for their use in the production of vinegar, vitamin C, and cellulose. The food substrate rich in carbohydrates, sugar, alcohols, and/or ethanol enables AAB to rapidly and incompletely oxidize these substrates into organic acids (acetic acid). However, AAB are not studied to the same extent as many other food-grade and industrially important microorganisms. Moreover, AAB are regarded as undesirable spoilers in alcoholic fermentation [31].

Kombucha from Central and East Asia is a beverage obtained by the fermentation of sweetened boiled tea with a mixed culture of yeasts and acetic acid bacteria. Other names for kombucha, or "tea fungus", include "fungus japonicus", "tee kwass", "tea kvass", "champignon de longue vie", "Indo-Japanese tea fungus", and "Manchurian mushroom" [32]. The microbiological composition of the tea fungus exhibits the symbiosis between bacteria and fungus. The main acetic acid bacteria found in the tea fungus are the following: *Acetobacter xylinum, A. xylinoides, A. acetic, A. pasteuriansu, Bacterium gluconicum*. Yeasts isolated from tea fungus include *Schizosaccharomyce pombe, Saccharomycodes ludwiggi, Kloeckera apiculate, Saccharomyces cerevisiae, Zygosaccharomyces bailii, Brettanomyces bruxellensis, B. lambicus, B. custersii, Candida* and *Pichia* species. The yeast cells convert sucrose into fructose and glucose and produce ethanol. Acetic acid bacteria (AAB) convert glucose to gluconic acid and fructose into acetic acid. Caffeine and related xanthines of the tea infusion stimulate the cellulose synthesis by the bacteria. Acetic acid stimulates the yeast to produce ethanol and ethanol which in turn stimulate AAB to produce acetic acid [33].

2.4. Alkaline Fermentation

Alkaline-fermented food products play an important role in the diet of people from Asia, Africa, and worldwide. Protein-rich foods are the main substrate that are acted upon primarily by *Bacillus* spp., but other secondary microorganisms such as LAB, staphylococci, and micrococci are also involved. Alkaline fermentation involves proteolysis that releases peptides and essential amino acids. Furthermore, amino acids are degraded into alkaline compounds such as ammonia that cause an increase in pH (8–10). Some of the common alkaline-fermented foods include *soumbala, ugha, bikalga,* and *ntoba mbodi* from Africa; as well as *kinema, natto,* and *thua nao* from Asia [34]. Species of *Bacillus* that are present, mostly in legume-based fermented foods, are *Bacillus amyloliquefaciens, B. circulans, B. coagulans, B. firmus, B. licheniformis, B. megaterium, B. pumilus, B. subtilis, B. subtilis* var. *natto,* and *B. thuringiensis,* whereas strains of *B. cereus* have been isolated from the fermentation of *Prosopis africana* seeds for the production of *okpehe* in Nigeria. Some strains of *B. subtilis* produce λ-polyglutamic acid (PGA), which is an amino acid polymer commonly present in Asian fermented soybean foods, giving the characteristic of a sticky texture to the product.

Soybean is one of the common substrates for traditional alkaline fermentation in East and Southeast Asia and in West Africa. The main microorganism for alkaline fermentation of non-salted soybean involves *Bacillus subtilis*. During fermentation, protease and amylase enzymes act upon protein and insoluble sugar, and therefore improve the nutritional value of fermented soybean products. Compared to the non-fermented counterpart, fermented soybeans are rich in isoflavone genestein and gamma-polyglutamic acid (PGA). Isoflavone genestein acts as a chemopreventive agent against cancer, while PGA acts as dietary fiber to reduce the cholesterol level in serum and improves efficacy of calcium absorption [35]. Soybean products can be either fermented by *Bacillus* spp. (mostly *Bacillus subtilis*) or by filamentous molds (mostly *Aspergillus, Mucor, Rhizopus*). Non-salted and sticky soybean products fermented by *Bacillus* spp. are concentrated in an imaginary triangle with three vertices lying each on Japan (*natto*), eastern Nepal and north-eastern India (*kinema*), and northern Thailand (*thua nao*), named as the "natto triangle" or renamed as the "kinema-natto-thuanao (KNT)-triangle". Traditional *Bacillus* fermented soybean products other than this include *chungkokjang* of Korea, *aakhune, bekang, hawaijar, peruyaan,* and *tungrymbai* of India, *pepok* of Myanmar, and *sieng* of Cambodia and Laos [10].

Natto is one of the most popular alkaline-fermented soybean products consumed widely in Japan, such that one Japanese consumes 760 g of natto per year. It is served along with rice as breakfast or as flavoring in dishes. The distinct features of *natto* include its unique odor, flavor, and notably stringy, mucous material on the surface of the soybean. The *Natto* preparation method includes cleaning, soaking, and cooking of the soybean followed by inoculating it with *B. subtilis* var. *natto* and fermentation at 40 to 45 °C for 18 to 20 h. The stringy material formed during fermentation is a polypeptide of glutamic acid and fructan produced by *B. subtilis* var. *natto*. *Natto* contains nattokinase, a polypeptide composed of a total of 27 amino acid residues with anticoagulant, fibrinolytic, and blood pressure-lowering effects, and antioxidant activity [36].

Thua nao, an alkaline-fermented soybean product, is a rich source of free amino acids and is used as a condiment in northern Thailand. Traditionally, it is prepared by fermenting the boiled soybean (boiled for 3–4 h) in bamboo baskets covered with banana leaves. The fermentation at ambient temperature for three days results in a brownish slimy substance with an ammonia odor and which is rich in free amino acids [37]. The dominant microflora of *thua nao* was found to be *Bacillus* spp., a Gram-positive, strict or facultative aerobe and endospore-forming bacteria [38]. Similar, *kinema* is an alkaline soybean fermented product that constitutes a large part of the diet of people living in eastern Nepal, and Darjeeling and Sikkim in India. Traditionally, *kinema* is prepared from clean soybeans soaked overnight, followed by cooking, crushing, wrapping in leaves and sackcloth, and fermenting at 25–35 °C for 1–3 days. It is an inexpensive source of nutrition containing (per kg; dry weight basis) 356–487 g protein, 161–249 g crude lipid, 274–296 g carbohydrate, and a number of vitamin B and minerals [39]. *Kinema* with a pungent ammonia smell, a slimy texture, and a short shelf-life, is similar to "*natto*" and "*thua nao*" with *Bacillus subtilis* as the dominant microorganisms. Compared to unfermented soybean, fermented *kinema* is found to be richer in essential fatty acids and better in protein quality and digestibility [40]. Another traditionally fermented soybean product that acts as a low-cost source of high protein food for the local people of Manipur, India is *Hawaijar*. It is similar to "*natto*" but with a dark brown color and a unique odor and taste. In research carried out by Jeyaram et al. [2], a *Bacillus subtilis* group comprising *B. subtilis* and *B. licheniformis*, and *B. cereus* and a *Staphylococcus* spp. group comprising *S. aureus* and *S. sciuri* were isolated from 41 "*Hawaijar*" samples collected from household preparations and markets of Manipur.

Tempe, a traditional soybean fermented product obtained through fermentation with *Rhizopus* spp., originates in Indonesia. During fermentation, different fungal enzymes including proteases, lipases, carbohydrases, and phyatses are produced that break down macromolecules into simpler compounds, thus partly solubilizing the cell walls and intracellular material. The final fermented product therefore has an increased nutritional quality and digestibility and the cottony mycelium binds the soybeans forming a compact cake. *Tempe* fermented by *Rhizopus microsporus* caused a reduction in the severity of diarrhea in piglets by inhibiting the adhesion of enterotoxigenic *Escherichia coli* to intestinal brush border cells [41]. Table 4 summarizes the common alkaline-fermented foods and beverages of Asia.

Table 4. Some of the common alkaline-fermented foods and beverages in Asia.

Country	Raw Materials	Local Name	Microorganism	References
Thailand	Soybean	Thua nao	Bacillus subtilis	[35]
India	Soybean	Hawaijar	Bacillus spp.	[2]
Japan	Soybean	Natto	Bacillus subtilis var. natto	[36]
Korea	Soybean	Cheonggukjang	Bacillus Subtilis	
Nepal	Soybean	Kinema	Bacillus subtilis	[40]

3. Conclusions and Outlook

In conclusion, Asia is well-known for its exotic traditionally fermented food and beverage products produced using a wide range of raw materials, microorganisms and fermentation processes. The indigenous methods of fermentation were aimed to preserve and balance the availability of food sources. Furthermore, many scientific research studies have exhibited promising and sustainable opportunities related to these traditionally fermented food products. The nutritional values of fermented foods are related to a unique group of microflora that may enhance health benefits directly through the interaction with the host or indirectly through metabolites synthesized during fermentation. The bioactive compounds and other interactions within fermented food can add novel flavors to food and impart potential health benefits. However, future studies need to be conducted in order to explore various aspects of fermented food products, such as the determination of biomarkers for fermented food health benefits, safety concerns related to these products, and the bioaccessiblity of microbial metabolites.

Funding: This research received no external funding.

Conflicts of Interest: The author declares no conflict of interest.

References

1. Bourdichon, F.; Casaregola, S.; Farrokh, C.; Frisvad, J.C.; Gerds, M.L.; Hammes, W.P.; Harnett, J.; Huys, G.; Laulund, S.; Ouwehand, A.; et al. Food Fermentations: Microorganisms with Technological Beneficial Use. *Int. J. Food Microbiol.* **2012**, *154*, 87–97. [CrossRef] [PubMed]
2. Jeyaram, K.; Singh, T.A.; Romi, W.; Devi, A.R.; Singh, W.M. Traditional Fermented Foods of Manipur. *Knowl. Creat. Diffus. Util.* **2009**, *8*, 115–121.
3. Nair, A.J. *Introduction to Biotechnology and Genetic Engineering*; Engineering Series; Infinity Science Press: Hingham, MA, USA, 2008.
4. Law, S.V.; Abu Bakar, F.; Mat Hashim, D.; Abdul Hamid, A. Popular Fermented Foods and Beverages in Southeast Asia. *Int. Food Res. J.* **2011**, *18*, 475–484.
5. Wilburn, J.R.; Ryan, E.P. *Fermented Foods in Health Promotion and Disease Prevention: An Overview*; Elsevier Inc.: Amsterdam, The Netherlands, 2016.
6. Hernández-Hernández, C.; López-Andrade, P.A.; Ramírez-Guillermo, M.A.; Guerra Ramírez, D.; Caballero Pérez, J.F. Evaluation of Different Fermentation Processes for Use by Small Cocoa Growers in Mexico. *Food Sci. Nutr.* **2016**, *4*, 690–695. [CrossRef] [PubMed]
7. Jayasekera, S.; Kaur, L.; Molan, A.L.; Garg, M.L.; Moughan, P.J. Effects of Season and Plantation on Phenolic Content of Unfermented and Fermented Sri Lankan Tea. *Food Chem.* **2014**, *152*, 546–551. [CrossRef] [PubMed]
8. Blandino, A.; Al-Aseeri, M.E.; Pandiella, S.S.; Cantero, D.; Webb, C. Cereal-Based Fermented Foods and Beverages. *Food Res. Int.* **2003**, *36*, 527–543. [CrossRef]
9. Tamang, J.P.; Thapa, N.; Bhalla, T.C.; Savitri. Ethnic Fermented Foods and Beverages of India. In *Ethnic Fermented Foods and Alcoholic Beverages of Asia*; Tamang, J.P., Ed.; Springer: New Delhi, India, 2016; pp. 17–72.
10. Hossain, M.; Kabir, Y. Ethnic Fermented Foods and Beverages of Bangladesh. In *Ethnic Fermented Foods and Alcoholic Beverages of Asia*; Tamang, J.P., Ed.; Springer: New Delhi, India, 2016; pp. 73–89.
11. Ekanayake, S. Ethnic Fermented Foods and Beverages of Sri Lanka. In *Ethnic Fermented Foods and Alcoholic Beverages of Asia*; Tamang, J.P., Ed.; Springer: New Delhi, India, 2016; pp. 139–150.
12. Karki, T.; Ojha, P.; Panta, O.P. Ethnic Fermented Foods of Nepal. In *Ethnic Fermented Foods and Alcoholic Beverages of Asia*; Tamang, J.P., Ed.; Springer: New Delhi, India, 2016; pp. 91–117.
13. Sanpamongkolchai, W. Ethnic Fermented Foods and Beverages of Thailand. In *Ethnic Fermented Foods and Alcoholic Beverages of Asia*; Tamang, J.P., Ed.; Springer: New Delhi, India, 2016; pp. 151–163.
14. Kitamura, Y.; Kusumoto, K.-I.; Oguma, T.; Nagai, T.; Furukawa, S.; Suzuki, C.; Satomi, M.; Magariyama, Y.; Takamine, K.; Tamaki, H. Ethnic Fermented Foods and Alcoholic Beverages of Japan. In *Ethnic Fermented Foods and Alcoholic Beverages of Asia*; Tamang, J.P., Ed.; Springer: New Delhi, India, 2016; pp. 193–236.
15. Dung, N.T.P.; Phong, H.X. Vietnamese Rice-Based Alcoholic Beverages. *Int. Food Res. J.* **2012**, *20*, 1035–1041.
16. Manosroi, A.; Ruksiriwanich, W.; Kietthanakorn, B.; Manosroi, W.; Manosroi, J. Relationship between Biological Activities and Bioactive Compounds in the Fermented Rice Sap. *Food Res. Int.* **2011**, *44*, 2757–2765. [CrossRef]
17. Sirisantimethakom, L.; Laopaiboon, L.; Danvirutai, P.; Laopaiboon, P. Volatile Compounds of a Traditional Thai Rice Wine. *Biotechnology* **2008**, *7*, 505–513.
18. Fernandez-Panchon, M.S.; Villano, D.; Troncoso, A.M.; Garcia-Parrilla, M.C. Antioxidant Activity of Phenolic Compounds: From in Vitro Results to in Vivo Evidence. *Crit. Rev. Food Sci. Nutr.* **2008**, *48*, 649–671. [CrossRef]
19. Harbourne, N.; Marete, E.; Jacquier, J.C.; O'Riordan, D. Stability of Phytochemicals as Sources of Anti-Inflammatory Nutraceuticals in Beverages—A Review. *Food Res. Int.* **2013**, *50*, 480–486. [CrossRef]
20. Pattanagul, P.; Pinthong, R.; Phianmongkhol, A. Review of Angkak Production (Monascus Purpureus). *Chiang Mai J. Sci.* **2007**, *34*, 319–328.
21. Pattanagul, P.; Pinthong, R.; Phianmongkhol, A.; Tharatha, S. Mevinolin, Citrinin and Pigments of Adlay Angkak Fermented by *Monascus* sp. *Int. J. Food Microbiol.* **2008**, *126*, 20–23. [CrossRef] [PubMed]

22. Somanah, J.; Bourdon, E.; Rondeau, P.; Bahorun, T.; Aruoma, O.I. Relationship between Fermented Papaya Preparation Supplementation, Erythrocyte Integrity and Antioxidant Status in Pre-Diabetics. *Food Chem. Toxicol.* **2014**, *65*, 12–17. [CrossRef] [PubMed]
23. Leroy, F.; De Vuyst, L. Lactic Acid Bacteria as Functional Starter Cultures for the Food Fermentation Industry. *Trends Food Sci. Technol.* **2004**, *15*, 67–78. [CrossRef]
24. Yonzan, H.; Tamang, J.P. Microbiology and Nutritional Value of Selroti, an Ethnic Fermented Cereal Food of the Himalayas. *Food Biotechnol.* **2010**, *24*, 227–247. [CrossRef]
25. Rhee, S.J.; Lee, J.E.; Lee, C.H. Importance of Lactic Acidbacteria in Asian Fermented Foods. *Microb. Cell Fact.* **2011**, *10* (Suppl. 1), S5. [CrossRef] [PubMed]
26. Quirós, A.; Ramos, M.; Muguerza, B.; Delgado, M.A.; Miguel, M.; Aleixandre, A.; Recio, I. Identification of Novel Antihypertensive Peptides in Milk Fermented with Enterococcus Faecalis. *Int. Dairy J.* **2007**, *17*, 33–41. [CrossRef]
27. Tamang, B.; Tamang, J.P. In situ fermentation dynamics during production of *gundruk* and *khalpi*, ethnic fermented vegetable products of the Himalayas. *Indian J. Microbiol.* **2010**, *50*, 93–98. [CrossRef]
28. Paludan-Müller, C.; Valyasevi, R.; Huss, H.H.; Gram, L. Genotypic and Phenotypic Characterization of Garlic-fermenting Lactic Acid Bacteria Isolated from Som-fak, a Thai Low-salt Fermented Fish Product. *J. Appl. Microbiol.* **2002**, *92*, 307–314. [CrossRef]
29. Ribas-Agustí, A.; Gratacós-Cubarsí, M.; Sárraga, C.; Guàrdia, M.D.; García-Regueiro, J.A.; Castellari, M. Stability of Phenolic Compounds in Dry Fermented Sausages added with Cocoa and Grape Seed Extracts. *LWT—Food Sci. Technol.* **2014**, *57*, 329–336. [CrossRef]
30. Pothakos, V.; Illeghems, K.; Laureys, D.; Spitaels, F.; Vandamme, P.; De Vuyst, L. Acetic Acid Bacteria in Fermented Food and Beverage Ecosystems. In *Acetic Acid Bacteria: Ecology and Physiology*; Matsushita, K., Toyama, H., Tonouchi, N., Okamoto-Kainuma, A., Eds.; Springer: Tokyo, Japan, 2016; pp. 73–99.
31. De Roos, J.; De Vuyst, L. Acetic Acid Bacteria in Fermented Foods and Beverages. *Curr. Opin. Biotechnol.* **2018**, *49*, 115–119. [CrossRef] [PubMed]
32. Aidoo, K.E.; Rob Nout, M.J.; Sarkar, P.K. Occurrence and Function of Yeasts in Asian Indigenous Fermented Foods. *FEMS Yeast Res.* **2006**, *6*, 30–39. [CrossRef] [PubMed]
33. Dufresne, C.; Farnworth, E. Tea, Kombucha, and Health: A Review. *Food Res. Int.* **2000**, *33*, 409–421. [CrossRef]
34. Ouoba, L.I.I. Traditional Alkaline Fermented Foods: Selection of Functional Bacillus Starter Cultures for Soumbala Production. In *Starter Cultures in Food Production*; John Wiley & Sons, Inc.: Chichester, UK; Hoboken, NJ, USA, 2017; pp. 370–383.
35. Inatsu, Y.; Nakamura, N.; Yuriko, Y.; Fushimi, T.; Watanasiritum, L.; Kawamoto, S. Characterization of Bacillus Subtilis Strains in Thua Nao, a Traditional Fermented Soybean Food in Northern Thailand. *Lett. Appl. Microbiol.* **2006**, *43*, 237–242. [CrossRef] [PubMed]
36. Mani, V.; Ming, L.C. Tempeh and Other Fermented Soybean Products Rich in Isoflavones. In *Fermented Foods in Health and Disease Prevention*; Elsevier Inc.: Amsterdam, The Netherlands, 2016.
37. Dajanta, K.; Apichartsrangkoon, A.; Chukeatirote, E.; Frazier, R.A. Free-Amino Acid Profiles of Thua Nao, a Thai Fermented Soybean. *Food Chem.* **2011**, *125*, 342–347. [CrossRef]
38. Petchkongkaew, A.; Taillandier, P.; Gasaluck, P.; Lebrihi, A. Isolation of *Bacillus* spp. from Thai Fermented Soybean (Thua-Nao): Screening for Aflatoxin B_1 and Ochratoxin A Detoxification. *J. Appl. Microbiol.* **2008**, *104*, 1495–1502. [CrossRef]
39. Moktan, B.; Saha, J.; Sarkar, P.K. Antioxidant Activities of Soybean as Affected by Bacillus-Fermentation to Kinema. *Food Res. Int.* **2008**, *41*, 586–593. [CrossRef]
40. Shrestha, A.K.; Noomhorm, A. Comparison of Physico-Chemical Properties of Biscuits Supplemented with Soy and Kinema Flours. *Int. J. Food Sci. Technol.* **2002**, *37*, 361–368. [CrossRef]
41. Roubos-van den Hil, P.J.; Nout, M.J.R.; van der Meulen, J.; Gruppen, H. Bioactivity of Tempe by Inhibiting Adhesion of ETEC to Intestinal Cells, as Influenced by Fermentation Substrates and Starter Pure Cultures. *Food Microbiol.* **2010**, *27*, 638–644. [CrossRef]

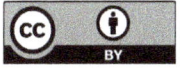

© 2019 by the author. Licensee MDPI, Basel, Switzerland. This article is an open access article distributed under the terms and conditions of the Creative Commons Attribution (CC BY) license (http://creativecommons.org/licenses/by/4.0/).

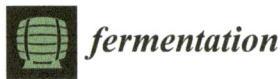

Article

Pesticide Residues and Stuck Fermentation in Wine: New Evidences Indicate the Urgent Need of Tailored Regulations

Pasquale Russo [1,2], Carmen Berbegal [1], Cristina De Ceglie [1], Francesco Grieco [3], Giuseppe Spano [1] and Vittorio Capozzi [1,2,*]

1. Dipartimento di Scienze Agrarie, degli Alimenti e dell'Ambiente, Università di Foggia, via Napoli 25, 71100 Foggia, Italy; pasquale.russo@unifg.it (P.R.); carmen.berbegal@unifg.it (C.B.); cristinadeceglie@libero.it (C.D.C.); giuseppe.spano@unifg.it (G.S.)
2. Promis Biotech srl, via Napoli 25, 71122 Foggia, Italy
3. Istituto di Scienze delle Produzioni Alimentari, Consiglio Nazionale delle Ricerche, Unità Operativa di Supporto di Lecce, 73100 Lecce, Italy; francesco.grieco@ispa.cnr.it
* Correspondence: vittorio.capozzi@unifg.it; Tel.: +39-0881-589303

Received: 25 December 2018; Accepted: 19 February 2019; Published: 24 February 2019

Abstract: For three consecutive years, an Italian winery in Apulia has dealt with sudden alcoholic stuck fermentation in the early stages of vinification process, i.e., typical defects addressable to bacterial spoilage. After a prescreening trial, we assessed, for the first time, the influence of the commercial fungicide preparation Ridomil Gold® (Combi Pepite), containing Metalaxyl-M (4.85%) and Folpet (40%) as active principles, on the growth of several yeasts (*Saccharomyces cerevisiae* and non-*Saccharomyces* spp.) and lactic acid bacteria of oenological interest. We also tested, separately and in combination, the effects of Metalaxyl-M and Folpet molecules on microbial growth both in culture media and in grape must. We recalled the attention on Folpet negative effect on yeasts, extending its inhibitory spectrum on non-*Saccharomyces* (e.g., *Candida* spp.). Moreover, we highlighted a synergic effect of Metalaxyl-M and Folpet used together and a possible inhibitory role of the fungicide excipients. Interestingly, we identified the autochthonous *S. cerevisiae* strain E4 as moderately resistant to the Folpet toxicity. Our findings clearly indicate the urgent need for integrating the screening procedures for admission of pesticides for use on wine grape with trials testing their effects on the physiology of protechnological microbes.

Keywords: pesticide; fungicide; wine; alcoholic fermentation; yeast; stuck fermentation

1. Introduction

Yeasts are responsible for the alcoholic fermentation process, i.e., the conversion of sugar into ethanol and CO_2, thus being the key player of the transformation of grape must into wine [1]. For this reason, among the different problems in wine production, the negative impacts on the fermentation process are of outstanding importance [2]. It is possible to distinguish two major types of fermentation problems: slow fermentative trends and stuck fermentation [3]. Due to the high risks of economic losses and of quality depreciation, the fermentation arrests represent one of the main challenges in winemaking [4,5]. Stuck fermentation is particularly hard to manage also because of the different possible physical, chemical and biological causes that make elaborate either the diagnosis and, the rectification too [4]. These considerations help explain the evidence suggesting that, despite considerable scientific advances and the existing panel of possible (bio)technological solutions, every year wine producers have to cope with consistent economic losses due to alcoholic stuck fermentation [6,7].

Grey mould (*Botrytis cinerea*), powdery mildew (*Erysiphe necator*) and downy mildew (*Plasmopara viticola*) are responsible for serious yield loss in the wine sector. They are the most damaging diseases of cultivated grapes (*Vitis vinifera*) worldwide, leading to severe injuries and resulting in significant commercial losses [8,9]. The use of several different fungicides to reduce the incidence of these viticulture pests can lead to the presence of organic residues, which must remain under the legal limit throughout the production process [10–14]. However, fungicides are often added without respecting the suppliers' prescription, thus causing the presence of organic residues in musts and wine over the legal limits. Moreover, chemical fungicides cannot be specific for the above pests and they can interfere with the biological function of other microbes, including protechnological organisms involved in food fermentations [15–17]. In fact, it has been demonstrated that, in some cases, fungicide residues can lead to modifications in the structure of the cellular membranes and in the metabolism of the yeast, affecting their activity during fermentation [18,19].

For three consecutive years, a winery in Apulia (southern Italy) has dealt with sudden fermentation arrests in the early stages of alcoholic fermentation. These sudden stucks in fermentation were difficult to justify and impossible to manage using classical (bio)technological approaches adopted by technical staff of the cellar (e.g., yeast nutrient integrations, addition of yeast starter cultures tailored for re-fermentation, variable concentration of free SO_2).

In order to identify possible physical, chemical or biological causes of observed stuck fermentations, we adopted a polyphasic approach suitable for considering some possible causes such as nutrients/oxygen starvation, high temperatures, low pH values and ethanol concentrations [4]. Among the other trials, we also preliminary tested the commercial pesticide formulations commonly used in the vineyard of this winery, for its capacity to inhibit the yeast starter cultures utilized in the cellar to promote the above stucked fermentations. As a result, a fungicide commercial preparation, Ridomil Gold® (Combi Pepite; Syngenta, USA), was found to provoke yeast growth inhibition. This commercial fungicide preparation contains Metalaxyl-M (4.85%) and Folpet (40%) as active principles, and it is commonly used in viticulture to fight the oomycete *Plasmopara viticola*, the causal agent of grapevine downy mildew.

In the present study, we examined the effect of this commercial fungicide preparation on the growth of *Saccharomyces* and non-*Saccharomyces* yeasts and lactic acid bacteria (LAB) of oenological interest, with the aim of determining its effects on the fermentation process. To the best of our knowledge, this is the first investigation aimed at assessing the impact of this commercial preparation on the growth/performance of the main protechnological microbes involved in winemaking.

2. Materials and Methods

2.1. Microbial Strains and Growth Conditions

Four commercial strains of *Saccharomyces cerevisiae*, namely Maurivin™ Elegance (Mauri Yeast Australia), Fervens® SLC (Dal Cin Spa, Concorezzo, Italy), Enartis Ferm SB (Enartis, Trecate, Italy), Lalvin RBS133 (Lallemand, Castel D'Azzano, Italy), and two indigenous *S. cerevisiae* strains (I6 and E4) previously isolated from Nero di Troia must [20], were used in this study. Autochthonous non-*Saccharomyces* yeast strains *Hanseniaspora guilliermondii* M105A31, *Hanseniospora uvarum* B05B29, *Issatchenkia orientalis* B05B2, *Issatchenkia terricola* B05B8, *Candida zemplinina* B05B6, *Torulaspora delbrueckii* B05B12, *Kluyveromyces thermotolerans* B05B32, *Metschnikowia pulcherrima* B05A22 and B05A36, and *Pichia fermentans* B05A29 and M105A3 were tested. These strains were isolated from Uva di Troia grape cultivar [21]. Flavia® (Lallemand), a *M. pulcherrima* strain, was isolated from a commercial preparation. Lactic acid bacteria used in this study were strains *Lactobacillus brevis* IOEB9809, *Lactobacillus hilgardii* CECT4786, *Lactobacillus plantarum* UFG44, *Leuconostoc mesenteroides* OT54, and *Pediococcus parvulus* UFG126. Yeasts and LAB were routinely grown at 30 °C on YPD and MRS (Oxoid, Basingstoke, UK), respectively.

2.2. Growth Curves in Media Contaminated with the Pesticide

Saccharomyces cerevisiae, non-*Saccharomyces* spp., and LAB strains were inoculated from cryo-conserved stocks (1:1000 v/v) in 30 mL of YPD or MRS, for yeasts and bacteria, respectively. After 24 h of incubation at 30 °C without shaking, cultures were diluted in fresh medium (1:100 v/v) artificially contaminated or not with 20.61 mg/L of Ridomil Gold® in order to achieve a final concentration of 1 mg/L of metalaxyl-M, corresponding to the legal EU limit in grapevine. Growth was monitored spectrophotometrically by measuring the optical density (OD_{600}) during 30 h of incubation at 30 °C in static conditions. Three replicates were performed for each assay.

2.3. Laboratory-Scale Vinification Assay

The laboratory scale vinifications were carried out by inoculating 150 mL of must from "Uva di Troia" grapes (sugars 230 g/L, pH 3.4). Commercial and autochthonous *S. cerevisiae* strains were inoculated at an initial concentration of about 1×10^7 CFU/mL in must supplemented with 20.61 mg/L Ridomil Gold®. The initial microbial concentration was determined by plate counting onto YPD agar, after incubation at 30 °C for 48 h. Control microvinifications were carried out in must without the addition of the pesticide. Fermentation progress was daily monitored by weight loss (indicative of CO_2 generation) measurement at 20 °C. The trials were performed in triplicate.

2.4. Laboratory-Scale Vinification Assay with Analytical Grade Standards

The commercial strain Lalvin RBS133, *S. cerevisiae* E4, *S. cerevisiae* I6 and twelve non-*Saccharomyces* strains were inoculated at an initial concentration of about 1×10^7 CFU/mL in 150 mL of must (from "Uva di Troia" grapes; sugars 230 g/L, pH 3.4) supplemented or not with the commercial pesticide or the analytical standard Folpet (8.24 mg/L) and Metalaxyl-M (1 mg/L) (Sigma Aldrich, St. Louis, MO, USA). Standards were added independently or in combination (8.24 mg/L Folpet and 1 mg/L Metalaxyl-M). A further control was the untreated and spontaneously fermented must. Microvinifications were carried out at 20 °C and monitored daily by weight loss. Experiments were performed in triplicate.

2.5. Laboratory-Scale Vinification Assay in Complex Microbial Ecosystem

In order to reproduce a complex microbial ecosystem like must fermentation, microvinification assays (performed at the same conditions as reported above) were repeated by using a mixed-fermentation approach, as detailed in Table 1. Non-*Saccharomyces* strains were divided into two panels, each including six strains, based on their resistance (panel R) or susceptibility (panel S) to the fungicide compounds. Both panels contained 1×10^7 CFU/mL of each strain. Three more resistant *S. cerevisiae* strains were independently co-inoculated with each panel at an initial concentration of 1×10^7 CFU/mL, as determined by plate counting. Samples were also contaminated with a mix of five oenological LAB (10^4 CFU/mL of each species). Microvinifications, including untreated must as control, were carried out at 20 °C and daily monitored by weight loss. Experiments were performed in triplicate.

Table 1. Strains of non-*Saccharomyces* and oenological lactic acid bacteria (LAB) co-inoculated with *Saccharomyces cerevisiae* strains in the laboratory-scale vinification assay in complex microbial ecosystem.

Non-*Saccharomyces*		Lactic Acid Bacteria
Panel S	Panel R	
I. orientalis B05B2	*P. fermentans* B05A29	*L. brevis* IOEB9809
M. pulcherrima B05A22	*P. fermentans* M105A3	*L. hilgardii* CECT4786
H. guillermondi M105A31	*C. zemplinina* B05B6	*L. plantarum* UFG44
H. uvarum B05B29	*T. delbrueckii* B05B12	*L. mesenteroides* OT54
M. pulcherrima B05A36	*I. terricola* B05B8	*P. parvulus* UFG126
K. thermotolerans B05B32	Flavia®	

2.6. Fungicide Residue Analysis

The analytical determinations of the fungicidal active principles were performed according to the European Standard Method EN 15662:2008 "Foods of plant origin—Determination of pesticide residues using GC-MS following acetonitrile extraction/partitioning and cleanup by dispersive SPE—QuEChERS-method" [22]. In particular, the analysis was performed using a GC/MS Agilent device (Little Falls, DE, USA) gas chromatograph 7890A, coupled with triple quadrupole spectrometry (7000C, Agilent). Pesticides were separated on an HP-5 ms UI capillary column from Agilent (0.25 mm i.d. × 30 m, 0.25 µm film thickness). The column was set at a constant flow rate of 1 mL min^{-1} using helium as carrier gas. The oven temperature was programmed as follows: the initial temperature was 60 °C, held for 1 min, increased to 120 °C at 40 °C/min, then ramped to 310 °C at 5 °C/min; the total run time was 40.5 min. The injector temperature was 280 °C and injection volume was 1 µL in splitless mode. The ion source and transfer line temperature was set at 280 °C. The data were processed with MassHunter software (B.07.00 Agilent). High purity pesticide analytical standards and internal standards were purchased from Sigma–Aldrich (Sigma Aldrich, St. Louis, MO, USA).

2.7. Statistical Analysis

Data were subjected to one-way analysis of variance (ANOVA). Pairwise comparison of treatment means was achieved by Tukey's procedure with a significance level of p values < 0.05, using the statistical software Past 3.0.

3. Results and Discussion

The aim of the present study was to investigate the causes of stuck fermentation detected for three consecutive years in the same winery. Initially, we adopted a polyphasic approach suitable to exclude some possible causes of stuck fermentation already described by other authors [4,23]. For these purposes, we studied the effects of nutrients/oxygen starvation, high temperatures, low pH values and ethanol concentrations on the same starter cultures utilized in the cellar to promote the alcoholic fermentation process. The obtained results indicated that none of the above parameters influenced, under the real fermentation conditions, the yeast starter growth [24].

Based on the above evidence, we decided to enlarge the scale of our investigation to assess the effects on fermentations of the pesticide sprayed on the grapes utilized for vinifications. The commercial fungicide routinely employed in the vineyard was the Ridomil Gold®, Combi Pepite (Syngenta). This pesticide, which contains Metalaxyl-M (4.85%) and Folpet (40%) as active principles, is commonly used in viticulture to fight the oomycete pathogen *Plasmopara viticola*, agent of the downy mildew in grapevine [25].

In a preliminary assay, we monitored the growth of *Saccharomyces* spp., non-*Saccharomyces* spp. and LAB in synthetic culture media (YPD and MRS for yeasts and LAB, respectively) supplemented with Ridomil Gold® (Combi Pepite). Currently, the EU limit in wine grapes for Metalaxyl-M and Folpet are 1 and 20 mg/L, respectively [14]. Therefore, based on the pesticide composition, containing Metalaxyl-M (4.85%) and Folpet (40%), the assays were performed by adding 20.61 mg/L of Ridomil Gold, an amount corresponding to 1 and 8.24 mg/L of Metalaxyl-M and Folpet, respectively.

As reported in Figure 1, the growth of *S. cerevisiae* was always lower in pesticide-enriched media when compared with the untreated control. In particular, the commercial strains Fermens and Elegance were mainly affected by the presence of Ridomil Gold (Figure 1). Interestingly, non-*Saccharomyces* strains showed a variable reduction in their growth rate in media with the pesticide formulation. For example, the growth of *H. uvarum*, *H. guillermondii*, *I. terricola*, *I. orientalis*, and some strains of *M. pulcherrima*, was completely inhibited in media containing Ridomil Gold [24], whereas *T. delbrueckii*, *P. fermentans*, *C. zemplinina*, and the commercial *M. pulcherrima* strains were more resistant at the same conditions. Interestingly, *T. delbrueckii* B05B12 seems to be more resistant than *S. cerevisiae* strains. Indeed, after a pre-adaptation time of about 24 h, the kinetics of growth of B05B12 did not seem to be influenced by the presence of the pesticide (Figure 1B). In contrast, contamination of Ridomil Gold in MRS broth did not affect the growth of any of the tested LAB (Figure 1C).

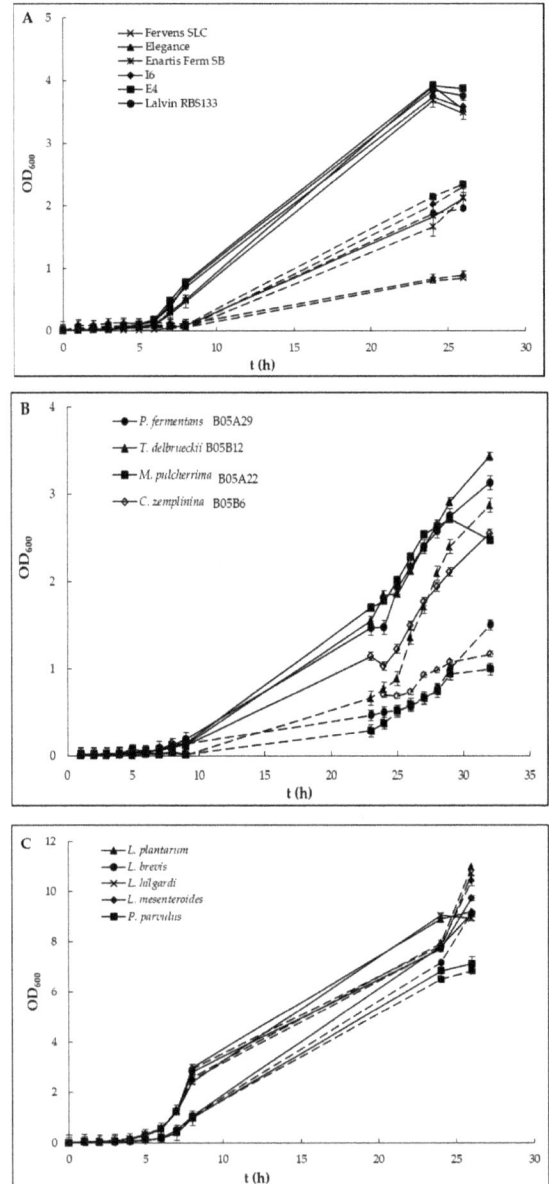

Figure 1. Growth of strains of *S. cerevisiae* (**A**), non-*Saccharomyces* (**B**), and LAB (**C**) inoculated in YPD (yeasts) and MRS (bacteria) supplemented (dashed lines) or not (continuous lines) with 20.6 mg/L of Ridomil Gold.

In a subsequent step, we monitored the fermentation process of grape must of the variety "Uva di Troia", artificially contaminated with the same concentration of Ridomil and inoculated with commercial and indigenous strains of *S. cerevisiae*. Using fungicide residue analysis, we verified that the concentration of active principles in the artificially contaminated sample corresponded to the dilution of quantities claimed in the product specification [24]. As shown in Figure 2, we found that, in the must without Ridomil the fermentation happened regularly, resulting in approximately 10% of weight reduction within two weeks. In contrast, when must was supplemented with the commercial formulation of pesticide, a slower and incomplete fermentation occurred, in all the assays, because the weight loss after 2 weeks was about 3% for all the investigated strains (Figure 2). These evidences strongly suggested that the presence of Ridomil was responsible for the stuck fermentation observed for three consecutive years in the winery.

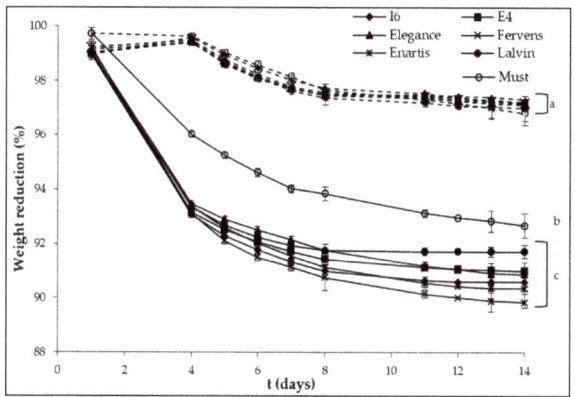

Figure 2. Microvinifications monitored for 14 days by weight reduction (%) of must not contaminated (dashed lines) or contaminated (continuous lines) with a Ridomil Gold® preparation containing 1 mg/L of Metalaxyl-M and inoculated with commercial and autochthonous *S. cerevisiae* strains. Sample "Must" was submitted to spontaneous fermentation. Different superscript letters indicate statistically significant differences ($p < 0.05$) in the weight reduction as determined by one-way analysis of variance (ANOVA).

In order to investigate if the stuck fermentation resulted from the specific action of the Ridomil active principles (i.e., Metalaxyl-M and Folpet) alone or in synergistic action, the analytical grade standards of these chemical compounds were also used as additive in the laboratory-scale vinification assays in comparison with the addition of the Ridomil itself. In order to challenge the interspecific and intraspecific variability in the tolerance to the excipients included in the commercial preparation twelve non-*Saccharomyces* and three *Saccharomyces* yeasts (namely, Lalvin RBS133, E4, and I6) were further investigated.

Samples were individually inoculated in must supplemented with: (i) nothing as control, (ii) Folpet (8.24 mg/L), (iii) Metalaxyl-M (1 mg/L), (iv) Folpet (8.24 mg/L) and Metalaxyl-M (1 mg/L), and (v) Ridomil Gold® (20.6 mg/L).

The results reported in Figure 3 and Supplementary Material S1 showed a great variability, indicating a different microbial susceptibility that could be either species- and/or strain-specific. In particular, when Ridomil was added to the must, the weight loss was always minimal compared with the other experimental conditions, and after 8 days the must was more than 98% of the initial weight (Figure 3 and Figure S1). A further reduction, detected during the second week corresponding to about 97% of the initial weight), was presumably associated with metabolic activities other than alcoholic fermentation. In general, no differences were observed in must untreated or supplemented with Metalaxyl-M. In contrast, Folpet strongly inhibited the fermentation, indicating that residuals of this molecule could be a serious concern during wine-making. Overall, three main different scenarios were observed. As model strains, we chose *T. delbrueckii* B05B12, *C. zemplinina* B05B6 and *S. cerevisiae* E4, and the corresponding profiles in the microvinification assays are summarized in

Figure 3. In general, no significant differences were found between samples supplemented with only Folpet or when Folpet was combined with Metalaxyl-M. This most abundant pattern was typical of twelve of the examined fermentations, including the spontaneous fermented control (Figure S1A–M). However, among the strains of this group, a markedly higher effect of the commercial Ridomil rather than Folpet or its combination with Metalaxyl-M was detected only for *Torulaspora delbrueckii* B05B12, and the commercial strains Flavia and Lalvin RBS133 (Figure 3A and Figure S1A–M). Only three samples, inoculated with *C. zemplinina* B05B6, *P. fermentans* B05A29, and *P. fermentans* M105A3, were characterized by a lower weight loss in must supplemented with Folpet and Metalaxyl-M than with only Folpet, suggesting a synergistic effect of both molecules (Figure 3B and Figure S1N–O). Intriguingly, the autochthonous *S. cerevisiae* E4 was the only strain unsusceptible to Folpet and Metalaxyl-M when added either independently or simultaneously to the must. Nonetheless, the same strain was unable to perform the alcoholic fermentation in samples contaminated with Ridomil Gold (Figure 3C), suggesting that different molecules, other than Folpet and Metalaxyl-M, could increase the effect of the commercial pesticide.

Interestingly, after about 2 weeks of the fermentation process, a thick gelatinous coating appeared on the surface of treated must, whereas, in untreated must, this coating was never detected (Figure 4). This finding clearly indicated that the arrest of fermentation turned the winemaking condition towards alterations of the wine, probably due to bacterial development.

On the basis of the biological information recently reported and related to the non-*Saccharomyces* biodiversity during the early steps of spontaneous alcoholic fermentation of "Nero di Troia" wines [26], we assessed the effect of the residual pesticide on the fermentation process in a more complex ecosystem resembling the microbial conditions of the must. "Uva di Troia" must was co-inoculated with each *S. cerevisiae* strain previously tested and two mixtures containing commercial and autochthonous non-*Saccharomyces* and LAB strains, as detailed in Table 1. According to the results obtained in the lab-scale vinification assay, the non-*Saccharomyces* yeasts were grouped into two panels, each containing six strains, based on their tolerance to Folpet: panel S including the most susceptible, and panel R including strains showing some resistance (Figure 5). A mix of LAB strains was also inoculated at a concentration of about 10^4 CFU/mL, according to their typical concentration in must [27]. The results showed that, in uncontaminated must, fermentation took place regularly, and a weight loss corresponding to 14 and 8% was detected (Figure 5A). As expected, alcoholic fermentation was faster in samples inoculated with the commercial *S. cerevisae* strains than with autochthonous yeasts. Interestingly, the weight reduction in presence of the panel R was higher, suggesting that non-*Saccharomyces* strains could differently affect the fermentation kinetics. In contrast, a stuck fermentation was always detected when must was supplemented with a Ridomil preparation containing 1 mg/L metalaxyl-M (Figure 5B). In general, no significant differences were detected, indicating that in the case of a complex microbial consortium the pesticide did not have an impact on the fermentation capabilities under these experimental conditions. However, samples inoculated with the autochthonous *S. cerevisiae* E4, which in our previous assay was resistant to Folpet, achieve the highest weight loss of about 5% after two weeks.

To the best of our knowledge, it is the first time that a commercial fungicide formulation recommended for control of pathogen on wine grapes and used within the legal limit was found responsible for grape stuck fermentation inoculated with *Saccharomyces* and non-*Saccharomyces* starter cultures. The potential of some pesticide formulations to induce fermentation arrests or to interact with the *S. cerevisiae* during fermentation has been already suggested [17,28]. In addition, the reported evidences testify that preliminary in vitro screenings are not always adequate to describe the possible negative effects of a commercial pesticide formulation on the fermentative performances of protechnological microbes. It was the case of *T. delbrueckii*, *P. fermentans*, *C. zemplinina*, and the commercial *M. pulcherrima* strain that displayed inhibitory behaviors under in vivo (in grape must) but not in vitro (culture media) trial conditions. Moreover, our results confirm a general scarce effect of fungicide preparation on malolactic bacteria [17]. Further studies will consider the effect of the commercial preparation on spoilage microbes of relevant interest in the wine industry (e.g., *Dekkera/Brettanomyces* [29–31]) and the application of specific timing management of microbial resources in vinification (e.g., coinoculation of yeasts and bacteria [32]).

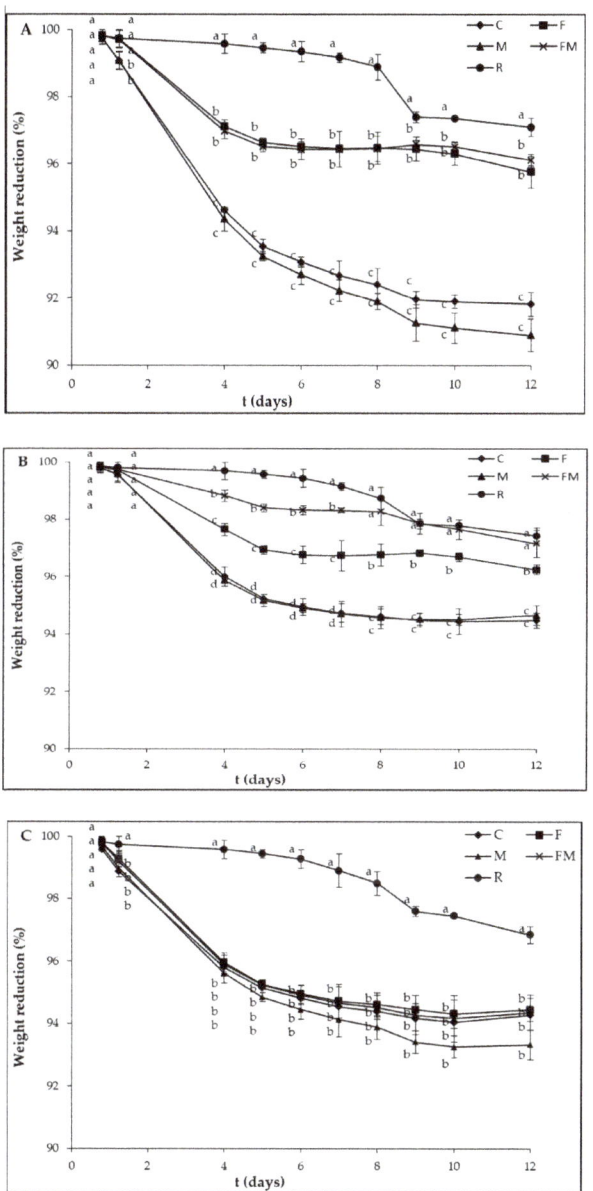

Figure 3. Microvinifications monitored for 12 days by weight reduction (%) performed by *T. delbrueckii* B05B12 (**A**), *C. zemplinina* B05B6 (**B**), and *S. cerevisiae* E4 (**C**) in untreated must (C), or supplemented with Folpet (8.24 g/L) (F), Metalaxyl-M (1 mg/L) (M), Folpet and Metalaxyl-M (FM), and Ridomil Gold® (R). Different superscript letters indicate statistically significant differences ($p < 0.05$) in the weight reduction as determined by one-way ANOVA.

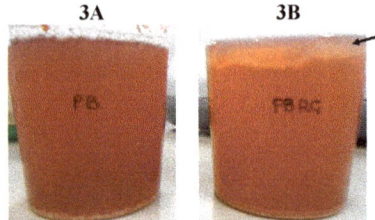

Figure 4. Appearance of the microvinification assay in must without (**A**) or supplemented (**B**) with 20.61 mg/L of Ridomil Gold® and inoculated with *S. cerevisiae* E4 after two weeks of fermentation. The arrow indicates the gelatinous coating on the surface of fermented must added with the pesticide.

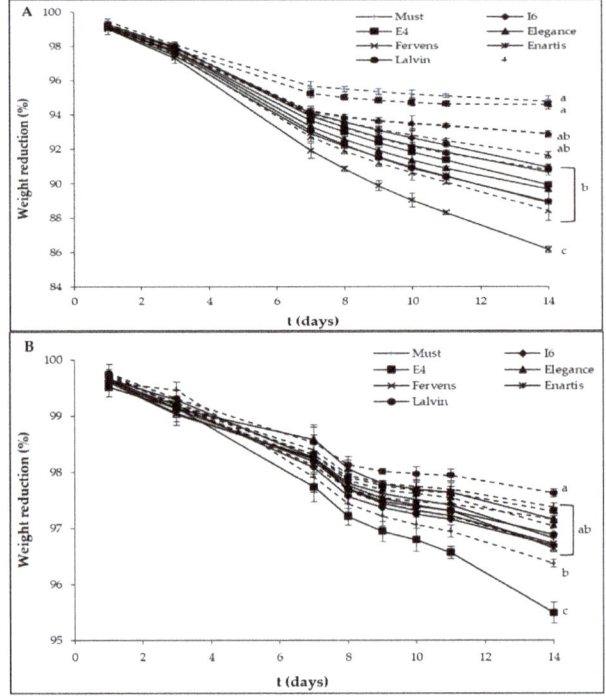

Figure 5. Microvinifications monitored for 14 days by weight reduction (%) of must not contaminated (**A**) or contaminated (**B**) with a Ridomil Gold® preparation containing 1 mg/L of Metalaxyl-M and inoculated with *S. cerevisiae* strains and panel S (susceptible non-*Saccharomyces* spp.—dashed lines), or panel R (resistant non-*Saccharomyces* spp.—continuous lines), and LAB. Different superscript letters indicate statistically significant differences ($p < 0.05$) in the weight reduction as determined by one-way ANOVA.

In the past, several molecules were investigated for their actions on wine microorganisms [17,33–35]. Considering the active principles present in Ridomil, different previous studies investigated the effects of Folpet on wine yeasts [17,36]. However, no data are available on the possible effects of Metalaxyl-M, whereas the effects of different pesticides used in the vineyard on oenological microbes have been described [37]. Our results generally confirmed the Folpet-induced reduction of fermentation activity of *S. cerevisiae* strains [17,35] but were unable to increase the fermentation rate of *Candida* spp. [17]. Furthermore, our findings underline the importance of testing the commercial formulation of fungicides rather than the single active principles and evaluating the effect in vivo rather than in vitro by direct assessment of pesticide formulation in the specific matrix.

4. Conclusions

In summary, for the first time, we have described the effect of two active agents present in the same commercial formulation on *Saccharomyces* and non-*Saccharomyces* species, underlining the possible increasing risks of fermentation arrests in case of pesticide formulation containing more active molecules. Furthermore, the fermentative behavior observed for the autochthonous strain *S. cerevisiae* E4 points out the possible inhibitory role of excipients included in the fungicide preparation and representing more than 50 % of the product. Our results shed new light on the need for an urgent tailored regulatory intervention on the mandatory characterization of pesticide formulations allowed for use on crops destined for the production of fermented food/beverages. All our findings were consistent with the recent literature on the influence of pesticides on other food-stuffs fermentations [17,19,38], and they clearly indicate the urgent need for integrating the screening procedures for admission of pesticides in agriculture with trials on the possible negative effects on protechnological microbes.

Supplementary Materials: Supplementary materials can be found at http://www.mdpi.com/2311-5637/5/1/23/s1. Figure S1: Weight reduction (%) of must in microvinification assays of twelve *Saccharomyces* and non-*Saccharomyces* strains inin untreated must (C), or supplemented with Folpet (8.24 g/L) (F), Metalaxyl-M (1 mg/L) (M), Folpet and Metalaxyl-M (FM), and Ridomil Gold® (R).

Author Contributions: conceptualization, P.R., F.G., G.S. and V.C.; methodology, P.R., C.B., C.D.C., F.G., G.S. and V.C.; investigation, P.R., C.B. and C.D.C.; resources, P.R., F.G., G.S. and V.C.; data curation, P.R., C.B., C.D.C., F.G., G.S. and V.C.; writing—original draft preparation, P.R.; writing—review and editing, P.R., F.G., G.S. and V.C.; supervision, F.G. and G.S.; project administration, F.G., G.S. and V.C.; funding acquisition, F.G., G.S. and V.C.

Funding: This work was supported in the framework of the projects named "Biotecnologie degli alimenti per l'innovazione e la competitività delle principali filiere regionali: estensione della conservabilità e aspetti funzionali (BiotecA)" and "Innovazioni di processo e di prodotto nel comparto dei vini spumanti da vitigni autoctoni pugliesi"—IPROVISP (Bando "Aiuti a Sostegno Cluster Tecnologici Regionali"; Project code VJBKVF4). Vittorio Capozzi was supported by 'Fondo di Sviluppo e Coesione 2007–2013—APQ Ricerca Regione Puglia "Programma regionale a sostegno della specializzazione intelligente e della sostenibilità sociale ed ambientale—FutureInResearch"'.

Conflicts of Interest: The authors declare no conflict of interest.

References

1. Berbegal, C.; Spano, G.; Tristezza, M.; Grieco, F.; Capozzi, V. Microbial Resources and Innovation in the Wine Production Sector. *S. Afr. J. Enol. Vitic.* **2017**, *38*, 156–166. [CrossRef]
2. Petruzzi, L.; Capozzi, V.; Berbegal, C.; Corbo, M.R.; Bevilacqua, A.; Spano, G.; Sinigaglia, M. Microbial Resources and Enological Significance: Opportunities and Benefits. *Front. Microbiol.* **2017**, *8*, 995. [CrossRef] [PubMed]
3. Blateyron, L.; Sablayrolles, J.M. Stuck and slow fermentations in enology: statistical study of causes and effectiveness of combined additions of oxygen and diammonium phosphate. *J. Biosci. Bioeng.* **2001**, *91*, 184–189. [CrossRef]
4. Bisson, L.F. Stuck and Sluggish Fermentations. *Am. J. Enol. Vitic.* **1999**, *50*, 107–119.
5. Capozzi, V.; Fragasso, M.; Romaniello, R.; Berbegal, C.; Russo, P.; Spano, G. Spontaneous Food Fermentations and Potential Risks for Human Health. *Fermentation* **2017**, *3*, 49. [CrossRef]
6. Maisonnave, P.; Sanchez, I.; Moine, V.; Dequin, S.; Galeote, V. Stuck fermentation: development of a synthetic stuck wine and study of a restart procedure. *Int. J. Food Microbiol.* **2013**, *163*, 239–247. [CrossRef] [PubMed]
7. Szopinska, A.; Christ, E.; Planchon, S.; König, H.; Evers, D.; Renaut, J. Stuck at work? Quantitative proteomics of environmental wine yeast strains reveals the natural mechanism of overcoming stuck fermentation. *Proteomics* **2016**, *16*, 593–608. [CrossRef] [PubMed]

8. Weng, K.; Li, Z.-Q.; Liu, R.-Q.; Wang, L.; Wang, Y.-J.; Xu, Y. Transcriptome of *Erysiphe necator*-infected *Vitis pseudoreticulata* leaves provides insight into grapevine resistance to powdery mildew. *Hortic. Res.* **2014**, *1*, 14049. [CrossRef] [PubMed]
9. Jacometti, M.A.; Wratten, S.D.; Walter, M. Review: Alternatives to synthetic fungicides for *Botrytis cinerea* management in vineyards. *Aust. J. Grape Wine Res.* **2010**, *16*, 154–172. [CrossRef]
10. Edder, P.; Ortelli, D.; Viret, O.; Cognard, E.; De Montmollin, A.; Zali, O. Control strategies against grey mould (*Botrytis cinerea* Pers.: Fr) and corresponding fungicide residues in grapes and wines. *Food Addit. Contam. Part Chem. Anal. Control Expo. Risk Assess.* **2009**, *26*, 719–725. [CrossRef] [PubMed]
11. Vaquero-Fernández, L.; Sanz-Asensio, J.; Fernández-Zurbano, P.; López-Alonso, M.; Martínez-Soria, M.-T. Determination of fungicide pyrimethanil in grapes, must, fermenting must and wine. *J. Sci. Food Agric.* **2013**, *93*, 1960–1966. [CrossRef] [PubMed]
12. Čuš, F.; Česnik, H.B.; Bolta, Š.V.; Gregorčič, A. Pesticide residues in grapes and during vinification process. *Food Control* **2010**, *21*, 1512–1518. [CrossRef]
13. González-Rodríguez, R.M.; Cancho-Grande, B.; Simal-Gándara, J. Decay of fungicide residues during vinification of white grapes harvested after the application of some new active substances against downy mildew. *Food Chem.* **2011**, *125*, 549–560. [CrossRef]
14. EU Pesticides Database—European Commission. Available online: http://ec.europa.eu/food/plant/pesticides/eu-pesticides-database/public/?event=homepage&language=EN (accessed on 22 December 2018).
15. Ochiai, N.; Fujimura, M.; Oshima, M.; Motoyama, T.; Ichiishi, A.; Yamada-Okabe, H.; Yamaguchi, I. Effects of iprodione and fludioxonil on glycerol synthesis and hyphal development in *Candida albicans*. *Biosci. Biotechnol. Biochem.* **2002**, *66*, 2209–2215. [CrossRef] [PubMed]
16. Calhelha, R.C.; Andrade, J.V.; Ferreira, I.C.; Estevinho, L.M. Toxicity effects of fungicide residues on the wine-producing process. *Food Microbiol.* **2006**, *23*, 393–398. [CrossRef] [PubMed]
17. Regueiro, J.; López-Fernández, O.; Rial-Otero, R.; Cancho-Grande, B.; Simal-Gándara, J. A review on the fermentation of foods and the residues of pesticides-biotransformation of pesticides and effects on fermentation and food quality. *Crit. Rev. Food Sci. Nutr.* **2015**, *55*, 839–863. [CrossRef] [PubMed]
18. González-Rodríguez, R.M.; González-Barreiro, C.; Rial-Otero, R.; Regueiro, J.; Torrado-Agrasar, A.; Martínez-Carballo, E.; Cancho-Grande, B. Influence of new fungicides—Metiram and pyraclostrobin—On *Saccharomyces cerevisiae* yeast growth and alcoholic fermentation course for wine production. *CyTA J. Food* **2011**, *9*, 329–334. [CrossRef]
19. Kong, Z.; Li, M.; An, J.; Chen, J.; Bao, Y.; Francis, F.; Dai, X. The fungicide triadimefon affects beer flavor and composition by influencing *Saccharomyces cerevisiae* metabolism. *Sci. Rep.* **2016**, *6*, 33552. [CrossRef] [PubMed]
20. Garofalo, C.; El Khoury, M.; Lucas, P.; Bely, M.; Russo, P.; Spano, G.; Capozzi, V. Autochthonous starter cultures and indigenous grape variety for regional wine production. *J. Appl. Microbiol.* **2015**, *118*, 1395–1408. [CrossRef] [PubMed]
21. Garofalo, C.; Tristezza, M.; Grieco, F.; Spano, G.; Capozzi, V. From grape berries to wine: population dynamics of cultivable yeasts associated to "Nero di Troia" autochthonous grape cultivar. *World J. Microbiol. Biotechnol.* **2016**, *32*, 59. [CrossRef] [PubMed]
22. Cunha, S.C.; Fernandes, J.O.; Alves, A.; Oliveira, M.B.P.P. Fast low-pressure gas chromatography–mass spectrometry method for the determination of multiple pesticides in grapes, musts and wines. *J. Chromatogr. A* **2009**, *1216*, 119–126. [CrossRef] [PubMed]
23. Malherbe, S.; Bauer, F.F.; Du Toit, M. Understanding problem fermentations—A review. *S. Afr. J. Enol. Vitic.* **2007**, *28*, 169–186. [CrossRef]
24. Russo, P.; Spano, G.; Capozzi, V. *Microbiological and Chemical Integrative Experimental Data*; Università di Foggia: Foggia, Italy, 2019; Material not intended for publication.
25. Čuš, F.; Česnik, H.B.; Bolta, Š.V.; Gregorčič, A. Pesticide residues and microbiological quality of bottled wines. *Food Control* **2010**, *21*, 150–154. [CrossRef]
26. Garofalo, C.; Russo, P.; Beneduce, L.; Massa, S.; Spano, G.; Capozzi, V. Non-*Saccharomyces* biodiversity in wine and the 'microbial terroir': A survey on Nero di Troia wine from the Apulian region, Italy. *Ann. Microbiol.* **2016**, *66*, 143–150. [CrossRef]

27. Lonvaud-Funel, A. Lactic acid bacteria in winemaking: Influence on sensorial and hygienic quality. In *Progress in Industrial Microbiology*; Ved Pal, S., Raymond, D.S., Eds.; Biotransformations; Elsevier: Amsterdam, The Netherlands, 2002; Volume 36, pp. 231–262.
28. Fatichenti, F.; Farris, G.A.; Deiana, P.; Cabras, P.; Meloni, M.; Pirisi, F.M. A preliminary investigation into the effect of *Saccharomyces cerevisiae* on pesticide concentration during fermentation. *Eur. J. Appl. Microbiol. Biotechnol.* **1983**, *18*, 323–325. [CrossRef]
29. Di Toro, M.R.; Capozzi, V.; Beneduce, L.; Alexandre, H.; Tristezza, M.; Durante, M.; Tufariello, M.; Grieco, F.; Spano, G. Intraspecific biodiversity and 'spoilage potential' of *Brettanomyces bruxellensis* in Apulian wines. *LWT Food Sci. Technol.* **2015**, *60*, 102–108. [CrossRef]
30. Capozzi, V.; Di Toro, M.R.; Grieco, F.; Michelotti, V.; Salma, M.; Lamontanara, A.; Russo, P.; Orrù, L.; Alexandre, H.; Spano, G. Viable But Not Culturable (VBNC) state of *Brettanomyces bruxellensis* in wine: New insights on molecular basis of VBNC behaviour using a transcriptomic approach. *Food Microbiol.* **2016**, *59*, 196–204. [CrossRef] [PubMed]
31. Berbegal, C.; Garofalo, C.; Russo, P.; Pati, S.; Capozzi, V.; Spano, G. Use of Autochthonous Yeasts and Bacteria in Order to Control *Brettanomyces bruxellensis* in Wine. *Fermentation* **2017**, *3*, 65. [CrossRef]
32. Tristezza, M.; di Feo, L.; Tufariello, M.; Grieco, F.; Capozzi, V.; Spano, G.; Mita, G.; Grieco, F. Simultaneous inoculation of yeasts and lactic acid bacteria: Effects on fermentation dynamics and chemical composition of Negroamaro wine. *LWT Food Sci. Technol.* **2016**, *66*, 406–412. [CrossRef]
33. Cabras, P.; Angioni, A.; Garau, V.L.; Melis, M.; Pirisi, F.M.; Minelli, E.V.; Cabitza, F.; Cubeddu, M. Fate of Some New Fungicides (Cyprodinil, Fludioxonil, Pyrimethanil, and Tebuconazole) from Vine to Wine. *J. Agric. Food Chem.* **1997**, *45*, 2708–2710. [CrossRef]
34. Cabras, P.; Angioni, A. Pesticide residues in grapes, wine, and their processing products. *J. Agric. Food Chem.* **2000**, *48*, 967–973. [CrossRef] [PubMed]
35. Oliva, J.; Cayuela, M.; Paya, P.; Martinez-Cacha, A.; Cámara, M.A.; Barba, A. Influence of fungicides on grape yeast content and its evolution in the fermentation. *Commun. Agric. Appl. Biol. Sci.* **2007**, *72*, 181–189. [PubMed]
36. Girond, S.; Blazy-Maugen, F.; Michel, G.; Bosch, M. Influence of some grapevine pesticides on yeasts and fermentation. *Revue Francaise d'Oenologie* **1989**, *29*, 14–22.
37. Sapis-domercq, S.; Bertrand, A.; Joyeux, A.; Lucmaret, V.; Sarre, C. Etude de l'influence des produits de traitement de la vigne sur la microflore des raisins et des vins. Experimentation 1977. Comparaison avec les résultats de 1976 et 1975. *OENO One* **1978**, *12*, 245–275. [CrossRef]
38. Đorđević, T.M.; Đurović-Pejčev, R.D. Dissipation of chlorpyrifos-methyl by *Saccharomyces cerevisiae* during wheat fermentation. *LWT Food Sci. Technol.* **2015**, *61*, 516–523. [CrossRef]

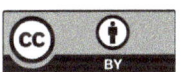

© 2019 by the authors. Licensee MDPI, Basel, Switzerland. This article is an open access article distributed under the terms and conditions of the Creative Commons Attribution (CC BY) license (http://creativecommons.org/licenses/by/4.0/).

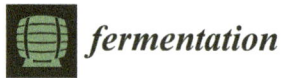

Article

Preliminary Screening of Growth and Viability of 10 Strains of *Bifidobacterium* spp.: Effect of Media Composition

Zuzana Matejčeková [1,*], Eva Vlková [2], Denisa Liptáková [3] and Ľubomír Valík [1]

1. Department of Nutrition and Food Quality Assessment, Faculty of Chemical and Food Technology, Slovak University of Technology, Bratislava, 812 37 Radlinského 9, Slovak Republic; lubomir.valik@stuba.sk
2. Department of Microbiology, Nutrition and Dietetics, Faculty of Agrobiology, Food and Natural Resources, Czech University of Life Sciences, Prague, 165 00 Kámycká 129, Czech Republic; vlkova@af.czu.cz
3. State Institute for Drug Control, Bratislava, 825 08 Kvetná 11, Slovak Republic; denisa.liptakova@sukl.sk
* Correspondence: zuzana.matejcekova@stuba.sk; Tel.: +421-2-59325-517

Received: 22 March 2019; Accepted: 24 April 2019; Published: 28 April 2019

Abstract: Lactic acid bacteria (LAB) alone or with special adjunct probiotic strains are inevitable for the preparation of specific functional foods. Moreover, because of their growth and metabolism, final products are preserved for a certain time. Thus, in this work, growth and metabolic activity of novel animal origin isolates and culture collection strains of *Bifidobacterium* spp. were investigated. The influence of milk media (reconstituted or ultra-high-temperature (UHT) milk), compared with synthetic modified Wilkins–Chalgren (WCH) broth under aerobic conditions was investigated. All tested bifidobacterial strains ($n = 10$) were grown well (1–2 log colony-forming units (CFU)/mL for 24 h at 37 °C) in all substrates and levels higher than 5 log CFU/mL remained during the cold storage period. Generally, different substrates determined almost the same maximal population densities (MPD) after 24 h that range within the average values of 8.96 ± 0.43 log CFU/mL, 8.87 ± 0.52 log CFU/mL, and 8.75 ± 0.54 log CFU/mL in reconstituted milk, UHT milk, and WCH broth, respectively. After 28 days of storage, the pH levels in milk media and broth were reduced to 4.50–5.60 and 4.60–4.90, respectively, representing a decrease of 0.8–2.13 units.

Keywords: *Bifidobacterium* spp.; fermentation; viability; shelf life; reconstituted milk

---

1. Introduction

Genus *Bifidobacterium* is one of the most beneficial probiotic microorganisms and one of the most predominant cultures in the human colon and breast-fed infants [1]. Until 2014, genus *Bifidobacterium* included 48 species and subspecies and this number is expected to increase [2]. *Bifidobacterium* is a genus of Gram-positive, catalase-negative, non-motile, and non-spore-forming bacteria. They are obligate, partly facultative anaerobes belonging to the Actinobacteria phylum, and are naturally predominant components of the intestinal microflora, presenting up to 20% of the fecal bacteria in adults and 80% in infants [3]. Properties of the strains belonging to the genus *Bifidobacterium* are host-dependent. The reported optimal temperature for the growth of human bifidobacterial strains is between 36 °C and 38 °C [2]; for species of animal origin, it is slightly higher (41–43 °C) and may be even as high as 49.5 °C, as shown for *B. thermacidophilum* [4]. There is also generally no growth below 20 °C with the exception of *B. psychroaerophylum*, whose growth was reported at temperatures as low as 8 °C [5]. The optimum pH for growth is in range of 6.0–7.0, which means that no growth takes place below 4.5 and above 8.5 [6].

Bifidobacteria exclusively catabolize hexoses through a characteristic metabolic pathway, involving fructose-6-phosphoketolase as the key enzyme, known as the fructose-6-phosphate pathway or the so-called bifid shunt. Generally, bifidobacteria preferably utilize mono- and disaccharides, while, within fermentation of glucose, some non-fermented strains were reported [7]. Some *Bifidobacterium* species are able to ferment lactose and are able to grow in milk such as *B. animalis* ssp. *lactis*. Thus, the fermentation ability of different substrates, including saccharides, their derivatives, and alcohols, is strain-specific [8]. Genus *Bifidobacterium* is a well-investigated group of beneficial microbes to human health. Within the food industry, if bifidobacteria are present in final products, due to the fact that they are obligate, partly facultative anaerobes, the presence of oxygen causes a decline in counts in final products during manufacture and storage. Therefore, it is important to study factors (e.g., presence of prebiotics, oxygen content in products) that affect the growth and viability of these beneficial bacteria in final products. Many factors were reported to affect the growth and survival of probiotic bacteria, including acid and hydrogen peroxide produced by yoghurt bacteria, oxygen content and oxygen permeation through the package, and the storage temperature [9,10]. In spite of the fact that bifidobacteria are considered to be strictly anaerobic, there are some species that are able to survive in the presence of oxygen [11]. *Bifidobacterium animalis* in a study of Lamoureux et al. [12] exhibited a high survival rate in prepared yoghurt, and inoculation of 7.4 log colony-forming units (CFU)/g was sufficient to obtain counts >6 log CFU/g after 28 days of cold storage at 4 °C. Havas et al. [13] reported that the fermentation process of soymilk resulted in a concentration of 8 log CFU/mL in all tested bifidobacteria after 8–12 h with all strains viable up to the end of fermentation (48 h). Maintaining the growth and viability of bifidobacteria in dairy products is a major challenge to dairy producers because of the inability of certain strains to grow and survive in milk. In order to investigate methods for improving the viability of bifidobacteria in commercial products, the viability status of these microorganisms was surveyed in real milk media and a model medium of synthetic broth. Thus, the influence of different kinds of substrates on the survival and acidification ability of *Bifidobacterium* spp. during cold storage was tested.

2. Materials and Methods

2.1. Bacterial Strains

The list of potentially probiotic bifidobacterial strains used in this study is shown in Table 1 and were provided by Prof. Vlková (Czech University of Life Sciences, Prague, Czech Republic).

The sub-cultivation of bifidobacteria was performed in serum bottles in Wilkins–Chalgren (WCH) broth (Oxoid, Czech Republic) according to Rada and Petr [14], supplemented with 5 g/L of soya peptone (Oxoid, Czech Republic), Tween-80 (1 mL/L; Biolofe, Italy), and Cysteine hydrochloride (0.5 g/L; Sigma–Aldrich Chemie GmbH, Switzerland) was added to act as an oxygen scavenger to provide a low redox potential. Bifidobacterial strains were stored in WCH broth added with glycerol (20 % v/v) before using it as an inoculum (stored at −20 °C).

Table 1. Origin of tested *Bifidobacterium* spp.

Bifidobacterium spp.	Origin
B. animalis subsp. lactis DSM 10140	Collection strain DSMZ
B. animalis subsp. animalis DSM 20104	Collection strain DSMZ
B. thermophilum DSM 20212	Collection strain DSMZ
B. animalis subsp. animalis 805 III2	Feces of calf
B. thermophilum 17 III2	Feces of calf
B. choerinum K1/1	Feces of goat
B. pseudolongum K4/4	Feces of goat
B. choerinum J14V	Feces of lamb
B. animalis subsp. animalis J5IIA	Feces of lamb
B. animalis subsp. animalis J3II	Feces of lamb

DSMZ—Deutsche Sammlung von Mikroorganismen und Zellkulturen, Germany.

2.2. Substrate Inoculation and Conditions of Cultivation

Milk medium was prepared from reconstituted milk (14% fat content; Bohemilk, Opocno, Czech Republic) according to the producer's instructions. Then, 100-mL aliquots were distributed into flasks, covered with lids, and boiled for 30 min. Subsequently, flasks were cooled down and tempered to 37 ± 0.5 °C. The standard suspension of the microorganisms was prepared by overnight incubation at 37 ± 0.5 °C and used in the individual experiments for inoculation of pre-tempered reconstituted milk, ultra-high-temperature (UHT) milk (1.5% fat content; Meggle, Bratislava, Slovakia), and modified WCH broth (added with soya peptone, Tween, and cysteine hydrochloride (see Section 2.1)) at an initial concentration of about 10^7 CFU/mL. The sterility of milk samples was regularly confirmed by the plating method prior to the inoculation. The fermentation process was carried out aerobically for 24 h at 37 ± 0.5 °C, followed by a storage period (6 ± 0.5 °C) within four weeks.

2.3. Enumeration of Bifidobacteria and Determination of Active Acidity

At appropriate time intervals, serial ten-fold dilutions of samples were prepared in a solution consisting of tryptone (5 g/L; Oxoid, Brno, Czech Republic), nutrient broth no. 2 (5 g/L; Oxoid, Brno, Czech Republic), yeast extract (2.5 g/L; Oxoid, Brno, Czech Republic), Tween-80 (0.5 mL/L), and cysteine hydrochloride (0.25 g/L). Bifidobacteria were cultivated and enumerated on a selective transoligosaccharide propionate medium with added mupirocin (TOS-MUP) (Merck, Darmstadt, Germany) recommended by the International Dairy Federation [15]. Petri dishes were cultivated at 37 ± 0.5 °C for 72 h under anaerobic conditions using anaerobic jars and an Anaerocult A system (Merck, Darmstadt, Germany).

After incubation, the grown colonies were counted, and the results were converted into colony-forming units per 1 mL of the sample. The pH values of the samples were monitored during fermentation and storage using a pH meter with a penetration electrode (Knick Portamess, Berlin, Germany) calibrated with buffers at pH 4.0, 7.0, and 10.0 (Fisher Scientific, UK).

2.4. Data Modeling

The growth parameters of studied bifidobacteria were fitted and calculated using the mechanistic model "DMFit" by Baranyi and Roberts [16], incorporated in the DMFit tools kindly provided by Dr. J. Baranyi (University of Debrecen, Debrecen, Hungary). The growth function of Baranyi and Roberts expressed in the explicit form was applied as follows:

$$y(t) = y_0 + \mu_{max} A(t) - \frac{1}{m} \ln\left(1 + \frac{e^{m\mu_{max}A(t)} - 1}{e^{m(y_{max}-y_0)}}\right) \tag{1}$$

where $y(t)$ is the natural logarithm of the cell concentration, y_0 is the natural logarithm of the cell concentration at $t = t_0$, t is time, t_0 is initial time of the growth, μ_{max} is the maximum specific growth rate, m is the curvature parameter to characterize the transition from the exponential phase (suggested values m running from 1 to 10), y_{max} is the natural logarithm of the maximum cell concentration, and $A(t)$ is the function that plays the role of a gradual delay in time.

$$A(t) = t + \frac{\ln\left(e^{-m\mu_{max}t} + e^{-h_0} - e^{-vt-h_0}\right)}{\mu_{max}} \tag{2}$$

where t is the time, h_0 is the dimensionless parameter quantifying the initial physiological state of the cells, and v is the curvature parameter for characterization of the transition to the exponential phase.

The criterion for "goodness of fit" is the percent variance accounted for (% V) and was calculated according to Equation (3) [17].

$$\% V = \left[1 - \frac{(1-r^2)(n-1)}{(n-n_T-1)}\right] \times 100 \qquad (3)$$

where n is number of observations in the dataset, n_T is the number of terms, and r^2 is the multiple regression coefficient.

Each experiment was performed in two separate trials. Statistical analyses were carried out using Microsoft Excel 2013 (Microsoft, Redmond, Washington, USA), with the addition of an analytical program Analyse-it (Analyse-it Software, Leeds, United Kingdom). The data were analyzed by the two-sided Tukey's post hoc test for means and Kruskal–Wallis test for medians of bifidobacteria as a group against substrates with a significance level of 0.05.

3. Results and Discussion

The most important factor in developing technology for the production of probiotic foodstuffs is growth and viability of applied strains. Although bifidobacteria are considered more susceptible to oxygen compared to lactobacilli due to their anaerobic nature, the oxygen sensitivity of microorganisms from the genus *Bifidobacterium* may, however, be strain-dependent [10]. Thus, the changes in viable cells of bifidobacteria under aerobic conditions during growth and survival of studied substrates were evaluated. Within 1% (v/v) concentration of tested bifidobacterial strains, an increase in bacterial counts under aerobic conditions of about 1–2 log CFU/mL (24 h, 37 °C) was observed. Generally, different substrates determined almost the same maximum population densities after 24 h, ranging within the average values of 8.96 ± 0.43 log CFU/mL (V = 4.8 %), 8.87 ± 0.52 log CFU/mL (V = 5.9 %), and 8.75 ± 0.54 log CFU/mL (V = 6.2 %) in reconstituted milk, UHT milk, and WCH broth, respectively. This statement was confirmed by Tukey's post hoc test, where mean differences were not significantly different ($p > 0.05$) within bifidobacteria and substrates tested.

High numbers of bifidobacteria may be attributed to the capability of tested microorganisms to detoxify oxygen as reported by Shimamura et al. [18]. Oxygen-tolerant bifidobacteria were also reported by various authors. Dave and Shah [19] found that bifidobacteria survived well (>10^5 CFU/g) over a 35-day period in yoghurt, regardless of the oxygen content and redox potential of the yoghurt. Shimakama et al. [20] also reported that *B. breve* strain Yakult needed about 12 h to reach the stationary phase with counts of 10^9 CFU/mL (from about 5×10^7 CFU/mL). *B. longum* and *B. bifidum* in soymilk in a study of Kamaly [21] increased their populations by about 1.8 and 2.4 log orders, whereas the corresponding values attained in reconstituted skimmed milk were 2.5 and 2.7 log CFU/mL.

All fermented milks can be considered a suitable food matrix for probiotic bacteria supplementation, and values of 6–7 log CFU/mL (or /g) at the expiration date of final products are reported as adequate for providing positive effects on health of consumers [22]. In our study, the behavior of microorganisms during storage was not significantly ($p > 0.05$) affected by the bifidobacterial strains and media used, as analyzed by the Kruskal–Wallis test (Table 2). Generally, no remarkable variations ($p > 0.05$) in modified WCH broth within 28 days were found (final concentration varied from 8.26 to 9.98 log CFU/mL at the end of the cold storage period) (Figure 1). This fact can be explained due to the presence of easily fermentable glucose, yeast extract, purines, pyrimidines, and amino acids supplying the nutritive elements required for the growth and survival of bifidobacteria. Counts of *B. adolescentis* Int57 in a study of Wu et al. [23] were also well maintained above 7 log CFU/mL after 168 h in modified de Man, Rogosa and Sharpe (MRS) medium. According to Maganha et al. [24], bifidobacteria may be better cultivated on artificial media (WCH broth) than in milk. However, these media are expensive for bifidobacteria multiplication, and the excessive growth of such bacteria may provide unpleasant flavors of final products. Thus, the improvement of the conditions for the growth of bifidobacteria in fermented milk may be obtained by the addition of a nitrogen source (milk powder) or of substances that reduce the redox potential of the food matrix. Therefore, the next part of this study details the behavior of bifidobacteria in milk media (reconstituted and UHT milk).

In reconstituted milk, a slight decrease in counts of bifidobacteria within the storage period was noted (0.12–0.81 log units), depending on the strain tested. Nonetheless, a clear significant decrease in the viability of B. thermophilum 17 III2 during the cold storage of fermented reconstituted milk was recorded (4.2 log CFU/mL; a fast decline was neither observed in UHT milk nor modified WCH broth. Despite the decline in levels of B. thermophilum 17 III2, the counts did not drop below the limit of 10^5 CFU/mL, the minimum level suggested by some authors [25]. Also, lactobacilli in 10 commercial fermented milks in a study of Gueimonde et al. [26] were well maintained above 10^5 CFU/mL during the cold storage period (30 days). In our study, in reconstituted fermented milk, a slight increase in counts of K1/1 isolate (0.034 log CFU/mL/h) within the storage period was observed, with almost the highest counts reached at the end of the cold storage phase (9.2 log CFU/mL). The positive effect of reconstituted milk on high densities of bifidobacteria within storage could be attributed to the compact matrix and the buffering capacity of fermented milk media [27]. Maganha et al. [24] also observed a positive effect of the addition of milk powder on levels of B. animalis subsp. lactis, where counts ranged from 6.03 to 6.61 log CFU/mL during storage within 21 days. Counts of Bifidobacterium spp. in UHT milk in our study ranged from 8.04 to 9.63 log CFU/mL (Table 2) after 24 h with increased values after 28 days in DSM 10140, K1/1, and J5IIA strains. In this medium, the fastest reduction in the J3II strain was observed (−0.026 log CFU/mL/h). Baron et al. [28] demonstrated that the survival of microorganisms from the genus Bifidobacterium spp. in fermented milks is strain-dependent, which is in agreement with our study. Considering the high heterogeneity of microorganisms, the composition of an ideal cultivation medium may vary. Currently, the origin of probiotics from the human gastrointestinal tract intended for human consumption is not an essential criterion. Zielińska and Kolozyn-Krajewska [29] showed that several microorganisms found in consumed food products do not originate from human hosts, e.g., B. animalis subsp. lactis and Saccharomyces cerevisiae var. boulardii.

Table 2. Parameters evaluating behavior of Bifidobacterium spp. during 28 days of cold storage (6 ± 1 °C).

Microorganism	Reconstituted Milk			Ultra-high-temperature Milk			Wilkins–Chalgren Broth		
	N_{24}	N_{end}	k_d	N_{24}	N_{end}	k_d	N_{24}	N_{end}	k_d
B. animalis subsp. lactis DSM 10140	9.15 *	8.72 *	−0.001 *	8.34 *	9.15 *	0.019 *	9.40 *	9.40 *	-
B. animalis subsp. lactis DSM 20104	8.79 *	7.98 *	−0.003 *	9.46 *	7.46 *	−0.002 *	9.79 *	9.98 *	0.001 *
B. thermophilum DSM 20212	8.01 *	7.91 *	−0.003 *	8.83 *	7.62 *	−0.002 *	8.00 *	8.45 *	0.001 *
B. animalis subsp. animalis 805 III2	9.32 *	9.18 *	0.001 *	8.59 *	8.15 *	−0.001 *	8.83 *	8.97 *	0.00 *
B. thermophilum 17 III2	9.28 *	5.04 *	−0.009 *	9.63 *	9.15 *	−0.004 *	9.90 *	9.93 *	-
B. choerinum K1/1	8.97 *	9.20 *	0.034 *	8.35 *	8.50 *	0.001 *	9.00 *	9.26 *	0.001 *
B. pseudolongum K4/4	8.82 *	8.61 *	−0.002 *	9.23 *	8.91 *	0.000 *	8.95 *	8.90 *	−0.001 *
B. choerinum J14V	9.32 *	8.74 *	−0.005 *	8.04 *	7.04 *	−0.001 *	8.92 *	8.85 *	−0.001 *
B. animalis subsp. animalis J5IIA	9.35 *	9.20 *	−0.001 *	8.76 *	9.34 *	0.012 *	8.43 *	8.26 *	−0.038 *
B. animalis subsp. animalis J3II	8.85 *	8.69 *	-	9.48 *	5.78 *	−0.026 *	8.47 *	8.98 *	0.004 *
Medians for all bifidobacteria	9.06 **	8.71 **	0.002 **	8.80 **	8.33 **	0.001 **	8.94 **	8.98 **	0.001 **

N_{24}—counts after 24 h of fermentation (log CFU/mL), N_{end}—counts after storage period (log CFU/mL), k_d—rate constant for decrease of counts (log CFU/mL/h). * Mean values were not significantly different ($p > 0.05$), as analyzed by two-sided Tukey's test; ** no significant differences among the medians within a column for bifidobacteria as a group confirmed by the Kruskal–Wallis test ($p > 0.05$).

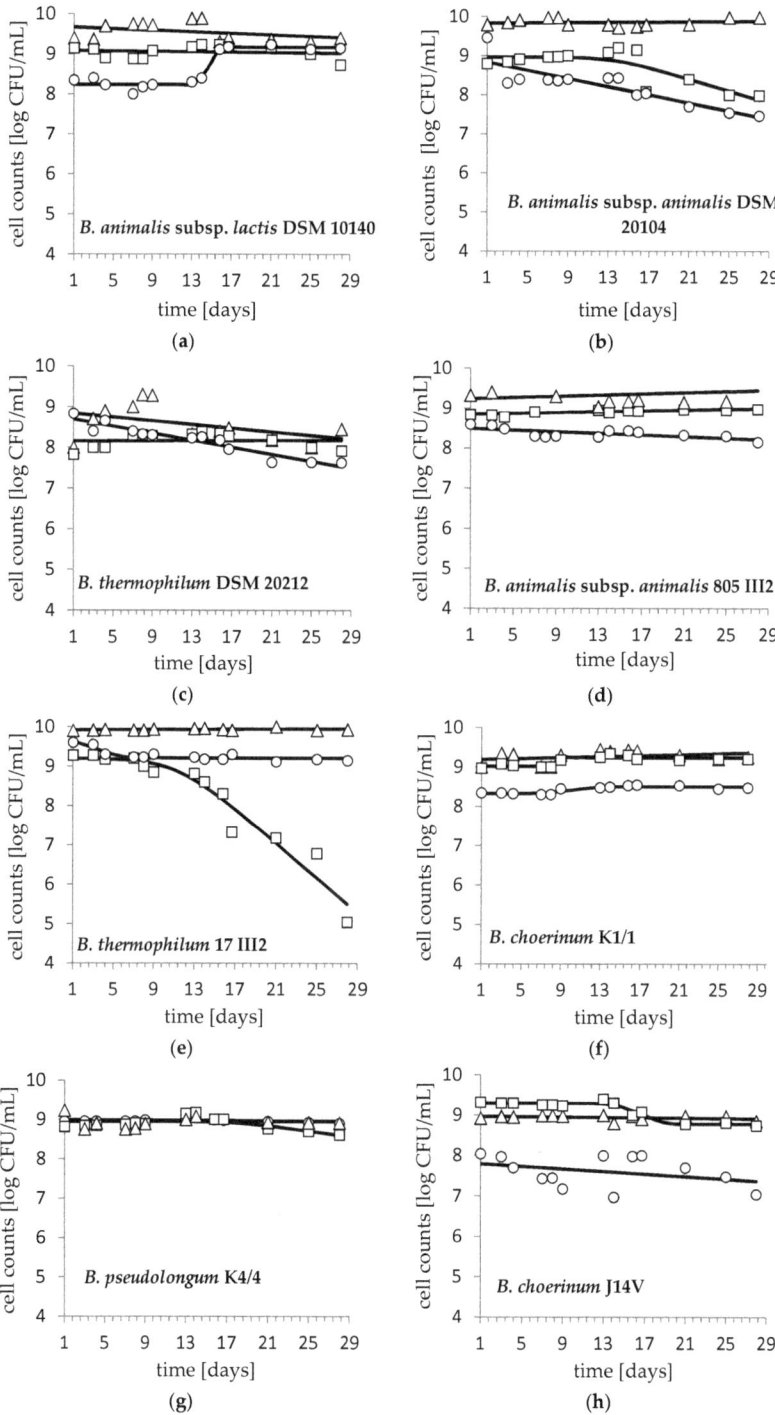

Figure 1. Cont.

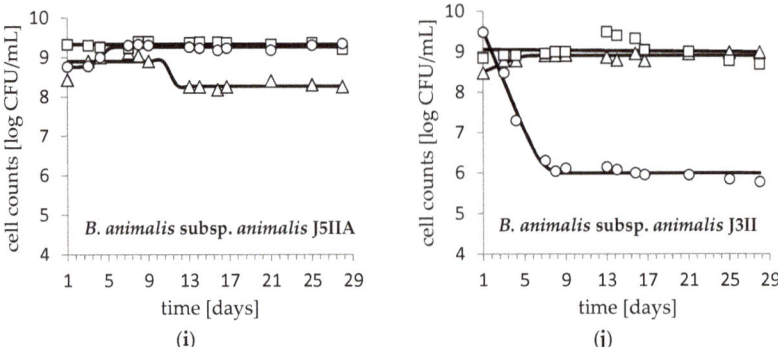

Figure 1. Survival of bifidobacteria in modified Wilkins–Chalgren (WCH) broth (△), fermented reconstituted milk (□), and fermented ultra-high-temperature (UHT) milk (○) in *B. animalis* subsp. *lactis* DSM 10140 (**a**) *B. animalis* subsp. *animalis* DSM 20104 (**b**) *B. thermophilum* DSM 20212 (**c**) *B. animalis* subsp. *animalis* 805 III2 (**d**) *B. thermophilum* 17 III2 (**e**) *B. choerinum* K1/1 (**f**) *B. pseudolongum* K4/4 (**g**) *B. choerinum* J14V (**h**) *B. animalis* subsp. *animalis* J5IIA (**i**) *B. animalis* subsp. *animalis* J3II (**j**) strains at 6 °C within four weeks.

To precisely evaluate the fermentation ability, in addition to measuring bacterial density, it is important to analyze the changes in the active acidity of growth media. Changes in media fermentation involve the conversion of carbohydrates to organic acids, resulting in a reduction in pH values. Rapid acidification is a priority for the development of starter cultures for fermented milk products [30]. Despite this fact, the growth and acid production of probiotic bacteria in milk is usually too slow to support an adequate fermentation process [9]. Matejčeková et al. [31] reported no significant changes in active acidity (0.00–0.24 units) in the *L. plantarum* HM1 strain during growth and multiplication in milk. Negligible acid production was also recorded in a study of Valík et al. [32] in *L. rhamnosus* GG in milk. This is not in agreement with our results, where, for all samples analyzed, there was a fast decrease in pH within 24 h (data not shown). The pH decrease during the fermentation of dairy products affects a number of aspects of the manufacturing process, including the quality, texture, and composition of the products [33]. In WCH broth, a decrease of about 1.58–2.13 units was recorded, with final pH varying from 4.60 to 4.90 after 28 days (Figure 2). These results are equivalent to the rate constant for a decrease of pH (k_{pH}) that varied from −0.08 to −0.14 h^{-1}. Krausova et al. [34] recorded a decrease in WCH broth from 6.40 to 4.69 on average in six lactobacilli strains and *B. bifidum* JKM. During the growth and multiplication at 37 °C, comparable pH changes of about 0.98–2.12 and 0.80–2.02 were observed in UHT and reconstituted milk, respectively. Similar observations in pH changes were reported in soymilk as an appropriate growth medium for lactic acid bacteria [21]. In our study, in UHT and reconstituted milk, final pH values at the end of 28 days of storage varied from 4.5 to 5.5 and from 4.5 to 5.4, respectively. Despite the low pH values that may affect the viability of tested microbes, bifidobacteria in our study survived in concentrations >5 log CFU/mL as stated previously. Regarding the shelf stability of samples analyzed, the post-acidification study is an important step since it reflects metabolic behavior of microbes used [35]. As seen in Figure 2, all samples analyzed followed an almost linear pattern within the storage period, except the DSM 20104 strain in reconstituted milk. In this strain, the pH reached after the fermentation (5.7) still decreased by about 0.19 units during storage with the rate of −0.05 h^{-1} (final counts = 7.98 log CFU/mL). The pH value of 4.5 is considered as a critical value in minimizing the outgrowth of the contaminating food spoilage and pathogenic bacteria. Generally, efficient acidification profiles are usually achieved when in co-culture [22]. Hence, further studies are required to assess the growth-promoting effects of co-cultivation with other strains of lactic acid bacteria used in dairy products.

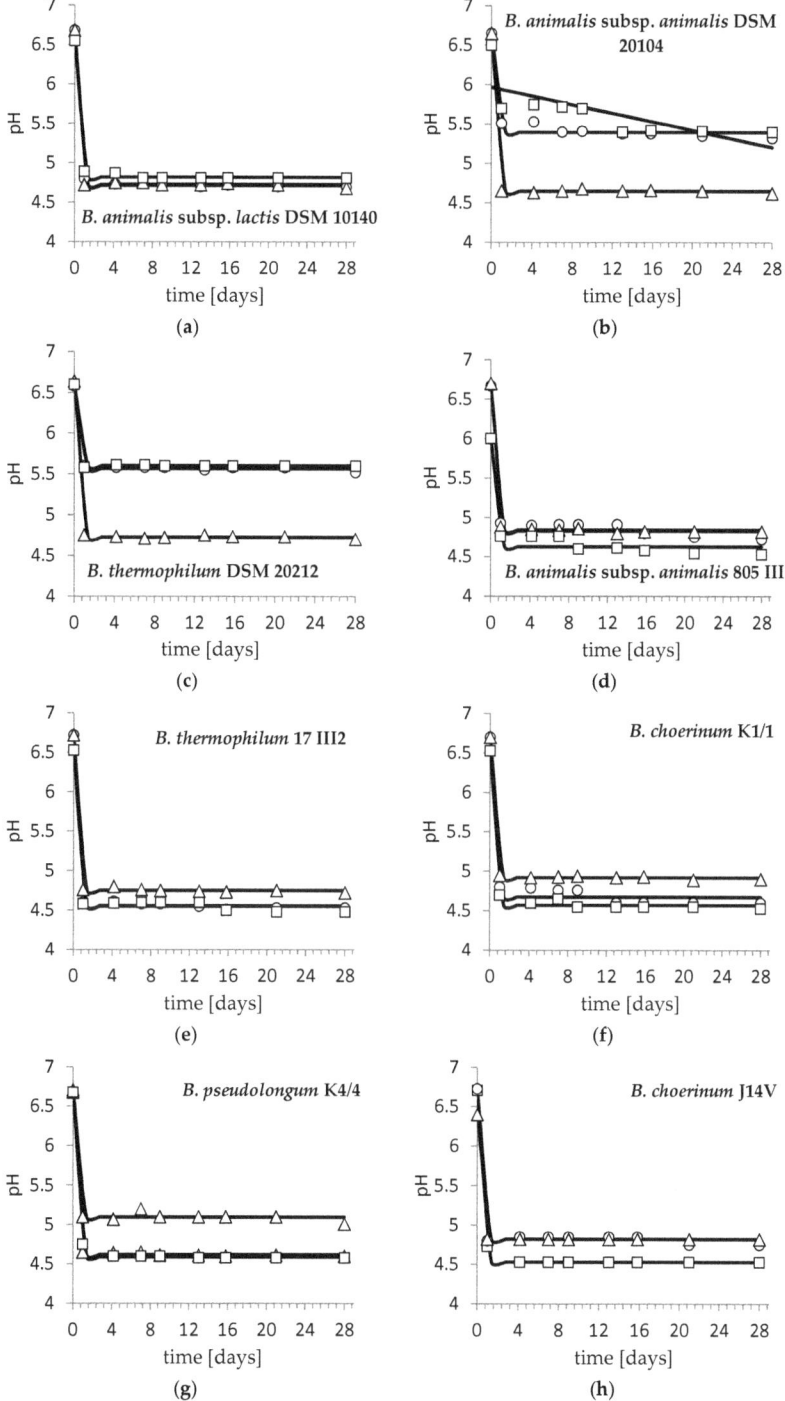

Figure 2. *Cont.*

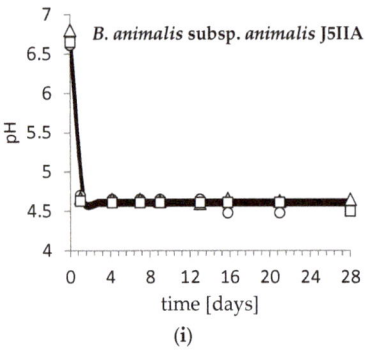
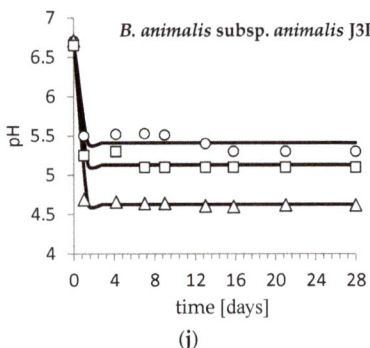

Figure 2. Changes in pH as a function of incubation time in modified WCH broth (Δ), fermented reconstituted milk (□), and fermented UHT milk (○) in *B. animalis* subsp. *lactis* DSM 10140 (**a**) *B. animalis* subsp. *animalis* DSM 20104 (**b**) *B. thermophilum* DSM 20212 (**c**) *B. animalis* subsp. *animalis* 805 III2 (**d**) *B. thermophilum* 17 III2 (**e**) *B. choerinum* K1/1 (**f**) *B. pseudolongum* K4/4 (**g**) *B. choerinum* J14V (**h**) *B. animalis* subsp. *animalis* J5IIA (**i**) *B. animalis* subsp. *animalis* J3II (**j**) strains at 6 °C within four weeks.

4. Conclusions

Since the growth responses of bifidobacteria are substrate- and oxygen-dependent, it is necessary to study the growth dynamic and viability of specific strains. Considering different types of products containing bifidobacteria available for Slovak consumers, experiments were realized in an artificial modified medium of WCH broth and in real media of reconstituted and ultra-pasteurized milk. Growth of 10 different species of bifidobacteria originating from the intestinal tract of animals and collection strains were studied in vitro under aerobic conditions. Maximal counts were generally achieved in WCH broth at the end of storage period at 6 °C for 28 days (from 8.26 to 9.98 log CFU/mL). The results of our study also indicate that the milk media used may serve as an excellent vehicle for dietary incorporation of *Bifidobacterium* cells. The results obtained may help optimize fermentation processes in dairy practice to provide reliable carriers of bifidobacteria for consumers.

Author Contributions: Z.M. performed the experiments, analyzed the data, and wrote the paper; E.V. provided microorganisms and set up the methodology; D.L. revised the manuscript and approved the final version for publication; L'.V. supervised and provided his expert comments within manuscript preparation.

Funding: This research was funded by the Scientific Grant Agency of the Ministry of Education of the Slovak Republic Vega No. 1/0363/19.

Acknowledgments: The authors are thankful to Marek Lelovský for English language corrections.

Conflicts of Interest: The authors declare no conflict of interest.

References

1. Awasti, N.; Tomar, S.K.; Pophaly, S.D.; Poonam, V.K.; Singh, T.P.; Anand, S. Probiotic and functional characterization of bifidobacteria of Indian human origin. *J. Appl. Microbiol.* **2015**, *120*, 1021–1032. [CrossRef] [PubMed]
2. Bunešová, V.; Vlková, E.; Rada, V.; Killer, J.; Musilova, S. Bifidobacteria from the gastrointestinal tract of animals: Differences and similarities. *Benefic. Microbes* **2014**, *5*, 377–388. [CrossRef]
3. Delcenserie, V.; Gavini, F.; Beerens, H.; Tresse, O.; Franssen, C.; Daube, G. Description of a new species, *Bifidobacterium crudilactis* sp. Nov., isolated from raw milk and raw milk cheeses. *Syst. Appl. Microbiol.* **2007**, *30*, 381–389. [CrossRef] [PubMed]
4. Dong, X.Z.; Xin, Y.H.; Jian, W.Y.; Liu, X.L.; Ling, D.W. *Bifidoabcterium thermacidophilum* sp. nov., isolated from an anaerobic digester. *Int. J. Syst. Evol. Microbiol.* **2000**, *50*, 119–125. [CrossRef]

5. Simpson, J.M.; Martineau, B.; Jones, W.E.; Ballam, J.M.; Mackie, R.I. Characterization of fecal bacterial populations in canines: Effects of age, breed and dietary fibre. *Microb. Ecol.* **2002**, *44*, 186–197. [CrossRef] [PubMed]
6. Jakubczak, A.; Stachelska, M.A.; Świstocka, R.; Lewandowski, W. The application of probiotic bacteria in the fermented vegetable cereal and meat products. *Polish J. Nat. Sci.* **2012**, *27*, 81–92.
7. Leahy, S.C.; Higgins, D.G.; Fitzgerald, G.F.; Sinderen, D. Getting better with bifidobacteria. *J Appl Microbiol* **2005**, *98*, 1303–1315. [PubMed]
8. Cronin, M.; Ventura, M.; Fitzgerald, G.F.; Sinderen, D. Progress in genomics, metabolism and biotechnology of bifidobacteria. *Int. J. Food Microbiol.* **2011**, *149*, 4–18. [CrossRef]
9. Shah, N.P. Probiotic bacteria: Selective enumeration and survival in dairy foods. *J. Dairy Sci.* **2000**, *83*, 894–907. [CrossRef]
10. Talwalkar, A.; Kailasapathy, K. The role of oxygen in the viability of probiotic bacteria with reference to *L. acidophilus* and *Bifidobacterium* spp. *Current Issues Int. Microbiol.* **2004**, *5*, 1–8.
11. Kawasaki, S.; Mimura, T.; Satoh, T.; Takeda, K.; Niimura, Y. Response of the microaerophilic *Bifidobacterium* species, *B. boum* and *B. thermophilum*, to oxygen. *Appl. Environ. Microbiol.* **2006**, *72*, 6854–6858. [CrossRef]
12. Lamoureux, L.; Roy, D.Y.; Gauthier, S.F. Production of oligosachcarides in yogurt containing bifidobacteria and yogurt cultures. *J. Dairy Sci.* **2002**, *85*, 1058–1069. [CrossRef]
13. Havas, P.; Kun, S.; Perger-Mészáros, I.; Rezseey-Szabó, J.M.; Nguyen, Q.D. Performances of new isolates of *Bifidobacterium* on fermentation of soymilk. *Acta Microbiol. et Imunol. Hung.* **2015**, *62*, 463–475. [CrossRef]
14. Rada, V.; Petr, J. A new selective medium for the isolation of glusoce non-fermenting bifidobacteria from hen caeca. *J. Microbiol. Methods* **2000**, *43*, 127–132. [CrossRef]
15. Vlková, E.; Salmonová, H.; Bunešová, V.; Geigerová, M.; Rada, V.; Musilová, Š. A new medium containing mupirocin, acetic acid, and norfloxacin for the selective cultivation of bifidobacteria. *Anaerobe* **2015**, *34*, 27–33. [CrossRef] [PubMed]
16. Baranyi, J.; Roberts, A.T. Mathematics of predictive food microbiology. *Int. J. Food Microbiol.* **1995**, *26*, 199–218. [CrossRef]
17. Davey, K.R. Modelling the combined effect of temperature and pH on the rate coefficient for bacterial growth. *Int. J. Food Microbiol.* **1994**, *23*, 295–303. [CrossRef]
18. Shimamura, S.; Abe, F.; Ishibashi, N.; Miyakawa, H.; Yaeshima, T.A.; Tomita, M. Relationship between oxygen sensitivity and oxygen metabolism of *Bifidobacterium* species. *J. Dairy Sci.* **1992**, *75*, 3296–3306. [CrossRef]
19. Dave, R.I.; Shah, N.P. Viability of yoghurt and probiotic bacteria in yoghurts made from commercial starter cultures. *Int. Dairy J.* **1997**, *7*, 31–41. [CrossRef]
20. Shimakama, Y.; Matsubara, S.; Yuki, N.; Ikeda, M.; Ishikawa, F. Evaluation of *Bifidobacterium breve* strain Yakult-fermented soymilk as a probiotic food. *Int. J. Food Microbiol.* **2003**, *81*, 131–136. [CrossRef]
21. Kamaly, K.M. Bifidobacteria fermentation of soybean milk. *Food Res. Int.* **1997**, *30*, 675–682. [CrossRef]
22. Matejčeková, Z.; Liptáková, D.; Valík, L'. Functional probiotic products based on fermented buckwheat with *Lactobacillus rhamnosus*. *LWT- Food Sci. Technol.* **2017**, *81*, 35–41. [CrossRef]
23. Wu, Q.Q.; You, H.J.; Ahn, H.J.; Kwon, B.; Ji, G.E. Changes in growth and survival of *Bifidobacterium* by coculture with *Propionibacterium* in soy milk, cow's milk, and modified MRS medium. *Int. J. Food Microbiol.* **2012**, *157*, 65–72. [CrossRef] [PubMed]
24. Maganha, L.C.; Rosim, R.; Corassin, C.H.; Cruz, A.G.; Faria, J.; Oliviera, C. Viability of probiotic bacteria in fermented skim milk produced with different levels of milk powder and sugar. *Int. J. Dairy Technol.* **2014**, *67*, 89–94. [CrossRef]
25. Matejčeková, Z.; Soltészová, F.; Ačai, P.; Liptáková, D.; Valík, L'. Application of *Lactobacillus plantarum* in functional products based on fermented buckwheat. *J. Food Sci.* **2018**, *83*, 1053–1062. [CrossRef] [PubMed]
26. Gueimonde, M.; Delgado, S.; Mayo, B.; Ruas-Madiedo, P.; Margolles, A.; Reyes-Gavilán, C.G. Viability and diversity of probiotic *Lactobacillus* and *Bifidobacterium* populations included in commercial fermented milks. *Food Res. Int.* **2004**, *37*, 839–850. [CrossRef]
27. Shaffie, G.; Mortazavian, A.M.; Mohammadifar, M.A.; Koushki, M.R.; Mohammadi, A.R.; Mohammadi, R. Combined effects of dry matter content, incubation temperature and final pH of fermentation on biochemical and microbiological characteristics of probiotic fermented milk. *Afr. J. Microbiol. Res.* **2010**, *4*, 1265–1274.
28. Barona, M.; Roy, D.; Vuillemard, J. Biochemical characteristics of fermented milk produced by mixed-cultures of lactic starters and bifidobacteria. *Lait* **2000**, *80*, 465–478. [CrossRef]

29. Zielińska, D.; Kolozyn-Krajewska, D. Food-origin lactic acid bacteria may exhibit probiotic properties: Review. *BioMed Res. Int.* **2018**, *3*, 1–15. [CrossRef]
30. Rathore, S.; Salmerón, I.; Pandiella, S. Production of potentially probiotic beverages using single and mixed cereal substrates fermented with lactic acid bacteria cultures. *Food Microbiol.* **2012**, *30*, 239–244. [CrossRef]
31. Matejčeková, Z.; Liptáková, D.; Spodniaková, S.; Valík, Ľ. Characterization of the growth of *Lactobacillus plantarum* in milk in dependence on temperature. *Acta. Chim. Slovaca.* **2016**, *9*, 104–108. [CrossRef]
32. Valík, Ľ.; Medveďová, A.; Liptáková, D. Characterization of the growth of *Lactobacillus rhamnosus* GG in milk at suboptimal temperature. *J. Food Nutr. Res.* **2008**, *47*, 60–67.
33. Liptáková, D.; Matejčeková, Z.; Valík, Ľ. Lactic acid bacteria and fermentation of cereals and pseudocereals. In *Fermentation Processes*; Jozala, A.F., Ed.; InTech: Rijeka, Croatia, 2017; Volume 3, pp. 223–254.
34. Krausova, G.; Rada, V.; Marsik, P.; Musilova, S.; Svejstil, R.; Drab, V.; Hyrslova, I.; Vlková, E. Impact of purified human milk oligosachcarides as a sole carbon source on the growth of lactobacilli in in vitro model. *Afr. J. Microbiol. Res.* **2015**, *9*, 565–571.
35. Campos, D.C.D.S.; Neves, L.T.B.C.; Flach, A.; Costa, L.A.M.A.; De Sousa, B.O. Post-acidification and evaluation of anthocyanins stability and antioxidant activity in acai fermented milk and yoghurts. *Rev. Bras. Frutic.* **2017**, *39*, 1–13. [CrossRef]

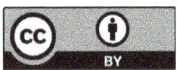

© 2019 by the authors. Licensee MDPI, Basel, Switzerland. This article is an open access article distributed under the terms and conditions of the Creative Commons Attribution (CC BY) license (http://creativecommons.org/licenses/by/4.0/).

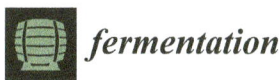

Article

Enterococci Isolated from Cypriot Green Table Olives as a New Source of Technological and Probiotic Properties

Dimitrios A. Anagnostopoulos, Despina Bozoudi and Dimitrios Tsaltas *

Department of Agricultural Sciences, Biotechnology and Food Science, Cyprus University of Technology, Limassol 3036, Cyprus; da.anagnostopoulos@edu.cut.ac.cy (D.A.A.); despoina.bozoudi@cut.ac.cy (D.B.)
* Correspondence: dimitris.tsaltas@cut.ac.cy; Tel.: +35-72-500-2545

Received: 9 May 2018; Accepted: 8 June 2018; Published: 20 June 2018

Abstract: Table olive is one of the main fermented vegetable worldwide and can be processed as treated or natural product. Lactic Acid Bacteria (LAB) are responsible for the fermentation of treated olives. The aim of this work was to study the technological characteristics and the potential probiotic properties of LAB isolated from Cypriot green table olives. This is the first comprehensive report on the isolation and characterization of LAB isolates retrieved from Cypriot green table olives. From a collection of 92 isolates from spontaneously fermenting green olives, 64 g positive isolates were firstly identified to genus level using biochemical tests, and secondly to species level using multiplex species specific polymerase chain reaction (PCR) amplifications of the *sodA* gene. Moreover, each of our isolates were tested for their technological and probiotics properties, as well as for their safety characteristics, using biochemical and molecular methods, in order to be used as starter cultures. Finally, to discriminate the most promising isolates on the base of their technological and probiotics properties, Principal component analysis was used. All the isolates were identified as *Enteroccocus faecium*, having interesting technological properties, while pathogenicity determinants were absent. Principal component analysis showed that some isolates had a combination of the tested parameters. These findings demonstrate that enteroccoci from Cypriot table olives should be considered as a new source of potential starter cultures for fermented products, having possibly promising technological and probiotic attributes.

Keywords: table olives; Lactic Acid Bacteria; *Enterococcus* spp.; technological characteristics; Probiotics

1. Introduction

Table olive is considered the most well-known among fermented foods in the Mediterranean area, constituting an important sector for the agro-industrial economy. Olives are the fruits produced by the olive tree (*Olea europea*). World production reach an average of 2.3 million tons per year, while the Mediterranean region is the main producer [1]. Most table olives (60% of the total production) are prepared following the Spanish-style (alkali treated green olives). However, nowadays, producers have displayed renewed and increasing interest in Greek-style fermentation, prepared with directly brined fruits [2]. Among the microorganisms involved in the fermentation process, Lactic Acid Bacteria (LAB) is the most essential and abundantly found group [3]. The development of LAB in the fermentation process, leads to a rapid acidification of the brine and a pH drop under 4.5 units [4].

LABs are gram-positive, non-spore forming bacteria. Due to the fact that they are facultative anaerobes they use their fermentative metabolism to provide energy. In general, LAB are a genetically diverse group of bacteria, encompassing rod-shaped bacteria such as lactobacilli, and cocci like streptococci, lactococci, enterococci, pediococci, or leuconostocs [5].

Enterococci are Gram-positive, non-spore forming, catalase negative, oxidase negative cocci and they occur singly, in pairs, or in chains. From a taxonomic point of view, the genus *Enterococcus* has been reviewed several times [6]. The genus includes more than 20 species, with *Enterococcus faecium* and *Enterococcus faecalis* being the most prevalent species in fermented foods [7]. It has been shown that those species produce bile salt hydrolases, presenting potential probiotic properties related to a reduction of serum cholesterol levels by promoting a higher excretion of deconjugated bile salts [8]. Due to their medium and/or high acid and salt tolerance, enterococci may be used in food fermentations as starter cultures, being responsible for the formation of unique flavors, as well as the production of enterocins [9]. Moreover, enterococci seem to be involved in table olive fermentation; In previous studies, it has been reported the presence of those LAB in Spanish-style green olives [9,10]. More specifically, Randazzo et al. [11] isolated four strains of enterococci belonging to the species *E. faecium, Enterococcus casseliflavus,* and *Enterococcus hirae* from naturally fermented green olives collected from different areas of Sicily region. Furthermore, it has been proposed the use of enterococci as starter culture for olive fermentation, because they play a crucial role at the initial stage of the process, due to their tolerance to high pH and salinity [11,12].

The aim of this work was to study the technological characteristics and the potential probiotic properties of LAB isolated from Cypriot green table olives, in order to discover new potential starter cultures for food fermentation industry.

2. Materials and Methods

2.1. Samples Collection

Nine samples of Cyprus variety of green cracked olives in round containers of 100 L brine (10%) fermenting for a period of one month (average temperature 25 °C), were collected from the company named "King of olives" in Agglisides, Cyprus, which is the largest producer of table olives in the country and processes olives from most production regions. This one month period was decided because in Cyprus the general practice is to consider the green cracked olives ready for consumption in 30 days of fermentation/debittering process. This is due to local market preferences of consuming green cracked olives while keeping their "freshness" or otherwise bitter taste. The brined samples were placed in sterile plastic containers and transported to the laboratory where they were stored in darkness at room temperature for analysis within 24 h. pH was measured in all nine samples by a portable pH meter (Hanna, UK).

2.2. Enumeration of Microorganisms

The samples were evaluated for their Total Viable Count (TVC), *Enterobacteriaceae*, LAB, yeasts, coliforms, *Micrococcaceae*, Gram-negative cocci and salt tolerant using the standard spread plate method after serial dilutions in saline water (0.85% (w/v)) (Table 1). More specifically, 10 g of table olives (flesh tissue) were transferred aseptically to stomacher bags with 90 mL saline solution (0.85% (w/v)) NaCl) and homogenized for 2 min using a Stomacher at 220 rpm for 2 min (Bug Mixer, Interscience, Saint Nom, France). Volumes of 0.1 mL or 1 mL (spread and pour plate, respectively) of serial dilutions in saline solution, were placed in petri dishes for enumeration of the microorganisms described. All samples were analyzed in triplicates.

Table 1. Microbiological media used for microflora enumeration.

Growth Media	Microorganisms	Method	Incubation Conditions
Plate Count Agar (PCA) (Merck, Darmstadt, Germany)	Total viable count	Spread plate	30 °C/72 h
De Man-Rogosa-Sharpe Agar (MRS) (Oxoid, Basingstoke, UK) + natamycin 4%	Lactic acid bacteria	Pour plate/Overlay	30 °C/72 h
M17 (Oxoid, Basingstoke, UK)	Lactic acid bacteria	Pour plate	37 °C/72 h
Sabouraud Agar (Oxoid, Basingstoke, UK)	Yeast and molds	Spread plate	25 °C/3 day
Violet Red Bile Glycose Agar (VRBGA) (BD, Sparks, MD, USA)	Enterobacteriaceae	Pour plate/Overlay	37 °C/24 h
Violet Red Bile Lactose Agar (VRBL) (Oxoid, Basingstoke, UK)	Coliforms	Pour plate/Overlay	30 °C/24 h
Baird Parker egg yolk tellurite (BPM) (Oxoid, Basingstoke, UK)	Micrococcaceae	Spread plate	37 °C/48 h
Nutrient Agar Crystal Violet (NACV) (Oxoid, Basingstoke, UK)	Gram cocci	Spread plate	21 °C/48 h
Mannitol Salt Agar (MSA) (Oxoid, Basingstoke, UK)	Salt resistant	Spread plate	30 °C/48 h

2.3. Isolation of LAB

Ten to 12 representative colonies according to their different morphological characteristics (size, shape, color etc.) were retrieved from De Man-Rogosa-Sharpe (MRS) agar Petri dishes with colony counts at the range of 30–300. Purity of the isolates was checked by streaking twice on MRS agar, followed by microscopic examination. Finally, stock cultures of purified isolates were stored at −80 °C in 20% (v/v) glycerol/MRS broth.

2.4. Physiological and Molecular Characterization of LAB Strains

The purified isolates were examined for Gram staining and catalase [13]. Gram-positive, catalase negative cocci were presumptively identified as LAB. Further classification was applied according to the biochemical criteria, such as growth at various temperatures (10 °C, 15 °C, and 45 °C), salt tolerance (2, 4, 6.5, 8% (w/v) NaCl), production of CO_2 from glucose as unique source of carbon and pH (9.6) [14,15].

The identification of the isolates at species level was achieved by applying molecular techniques by multiplex PCR amplifications of the *sodA* gene [16]. Three PCR master mixes consisting of different primer sets for each species were prepared (Table 2); Group 1 was *Enterococcus durans*, *E. faecalis*, *E. faecium*; group 2 was *E. casseliflavus*, *Enterococcus gallinarum*; group 3 was *E. hirae*. PCR reactions contained 2.5 µL template DNA (10 ng), 1× PCR reaction buffer, 0.2 mM of each deoxynucleotide triphosphate (dNTP), 3 mM $MgCl_2$, 16 µM of each primer, 2.5 U of Kappa Hot Start DNA polymerase (KAPPA Biosystems), and distilled water was added to a final volume of 22.5 µL. Following an initial denaturation at 95 °C for 4 min, products were amplified by 35 cycles of denaturation at 95 °C for 30 s, annealing at 55 °C for Group 1, 57 °C for Group 2 and 60 °C for Group 3 for 1 min, and elongation at 72 °C for 1 min. Finally, amplification was followed by a final extension at 72 °C for 7 min. Eight µL of PCR product was electrophorized on a 1.2% agarose gel, 1× TAE (Tris-acetate-EDTA), stained with SYBR™ Safe DNA Gel Stain (Invitrogen, Carlsbad, CA, USA) and visualized under UV light. A 100 bp DNA ladder (Nippon Genetics) was used as marker.

Table 2. Polymerase chain reaction (PCR) primers, products, and reference strains.

Strain	Primer	Sequence (5′–3′)	Product Size (bp)
E. durans ATCC19432	DU1 DU2	CCTACTGATATTAAGACAGCG TAATCCTAAGATAGGTGTTTG	295
E. faecalis ATCC19433	FL1 FL2	ACTTATGTGACTAACTTAACC TAATGGTGAATCTTGGTTTGG	360
E. faecium ATCC19434	FM1 FM2	GAAAAAACAATAGAAGAATTAT TGCTTTTTTGAATTCTTCTTTA	215
E. casseliflavus ATCC25788	CA1 CA2	TCCTGAATTAGGTGAAAAAAC GCTAGTTTACCGTCTTTAACG	288
E. gallinarum ATCC49673	GA1 GA2	TTACTTGCTGATTTTGATTCG TGAATTCTTCTTTGAAATCAG	173
E. hirae ATCC 8043	HI1 HI2	CTTTCTGATATGGATGCTGTC TAAATTCTTCCTTAAATGTTG	187

2.5. Technological Characteristics

2.5.1. Acidification Activity

Acidification activity of the *Enterococcus* isolates was tested according to Fuka et al. [17]. In particular, tubes containing 10 mL of sterile skimmed milk (D 10% (w/v); Oxoid) were inoculated with fresh overnight cultures (1% (v/v)) and incubated at 37 °C. The pH value was determined after incubation for 0, 6 and 24 h using a pH meter (Hanna instruments). The analysis was carried out in triplicate. A non-inoculated skim milk was used as negative control. The acidification rate was calculated as $\Delta pH = pH_{(0h)} - pH$ (6 h or 24 h respectively).

2.5.2. Proteolytic Activity

For the determination of proteolytic activity, 2 µL of fresh overnight cultures (10^8 cfu/mL) were spotted on the surface of a skim milk agar (10% (w/v) skim milk, 2% (w/v) agar, Oxoid), and were incubated at 37 °C from 2 to 4 days [18]. The results were considered as positive when a clear zone was formed around the colonies. The analysis was performed in triplicate.

2.5.3. Lipolytic Activity

For the determination of lipolytic activity, a loopful of fresh culture (24 h) was placed on tributyrin agar (Oxoid) and was incubated at 37 °C for 4 days [19]. The results were considered as positive when a clear zone appeared around the colonies. The analysis was repeated three times.

2.5.4. Exopolysaccharide Production (EPS)

EPS production was evaluated with ruthenium red staining method in ruthenium milk agar (0.5% yeast extract, 10% skim milk powder, 1% sucrose, 1.6% agar, 0.08 g/L ruthenium red) [20]. The coagulated cultures were considered as EPS-positive when a white loop was formed after incubation at 37 °C for 24 h. The analysis was conducted in triplicate.

2.5.5. β-Glucosidase Activity

β-glucosidase activity was determined using X-Gluc-5-bromo-4-chloro-3-indolyl-β-D-glucopyranoside (Sigma, Saint Louis, MO, USA) as substrate. The test was conducted by spreading 0.2 mL of a N,N-dimethyl formamide solution to a final concentration of 0.3% (w/v) X-Gluc on MRS agar. The plates were left to dry for 3 h in darkness, and were incubated at 37 °C for 48 h after the inoculation (2 µL) [21]. Isolates producing β-glucosidase were recognized when the colony was colored blue. The analysis was repeated three times.

2.5.6. Catabolism of Citric Acid

The determination of catabolism of citric acid was performed by growth in Simmons Citrate Agar (Oxoid), which contains citric acid as the only carbon source. Freshly prepared cultures were inoculated by spread to the medium and the plates were incubated at 37 °C for 7 days. Results were considered positive when colonies turned the color of the substrate from green to blue, otherwise the test was considered as negative. The analysis was performed in triplicates.

2.6. Pathogenicity

2.6.1. Hemolytic Activity

Freshly prepared cultures were inoculated by spread on Columbia Agar Base (Oxoid), supplemented with 5% (v/v) horse blood and incubated at 37 °C for 24 h. Hemolytic activity was characterized "α" when a green zone was formed round the colonies, "β" when clear zones were created around colonies, and "γ" when no zones were appeared around colonies [17]. The analysis was repeated in triplicates.

2.6.2. DNAse Production

Screening for DNAse production was held according to Ribeiro et al. [22]. The tested strains were grown at 37 °C in MRS broth overnight. A loopful of freshly prepared cultures was spotted on DNAse agar (Oxoid) and a few drops of 1 N HCl were added onto the colony, after incubation for 24 h at 37 °C. Production of DNAse was indicated when a clear zone appeared around the colonies. The analysis was repeated three times.

2.6.3. Virulence Activity Using Genotypic Tests

All the selected strains were checked for the presence of genes encoding virulence, antibiotic resistance and amino acid decarboxylase activity [23,24]. DNA was extracted using Bacterial DNA kit (Macherey-Nagel, Duren, Germany) according to the manufacturer's instructions, following by amplifications of genes described in Table 3 using specific primers. PCR reactions contained 1 μL template DNA (10 ng), 1× PCR reaction buffer, 0.2 mM of each dNTP, 1.5 mM $MgCl_2$, 16 μM of each primer, 1 U of Kappa Taq DNA polymerase (KAPPA Biosystems), and distilled water was added to a final volume of 20 μL. Following an initial denaturation at 95 °C for 4 min, products were amplified by 30 cycles of denaturation at 95 °C for 30 s, annealing of each primer for 30 s, and elongation at 72 °C for 1 min. Finally, amplification was followed by a final extension at 72 °C for 7 min. Eight μL of PCR product was electrophorized on a 1.2% agarose gel, 1× TAE (Tris-acetate-EDTA), stained with SYBR™ Safe DNA Gel Stain (Invitrogen, Carlsbad, CA, USA) and visualized under UV light. A 100 bp DNA ladder (Nippon Genetics) was used as marker. The DNA of the reference strain E. faecium ATCC 29212 was used as positive control in the corresponding PCR reactions.

Table 3. List of primers used for the amplification of pathogenicity related genes.

Target Gene	Primer Sequence	Annealing Temperature (°C)	Fragment Size (bp)	Reference
Aggregation substance (asa1)	GCACGCTATTACGAACTATGA TAAGAAAGAACATCACCACGA	50	375	[25]
Adhesion of collagen protein (ace)	GAATTGAGCAAAAGTTCAATCG GTCTGTCTTTTCACTTGTTTC	48	1008	[26]
Cytolysin (cylA)	ACTCGGGGATTGATAGGC GCTGCTAAAGCTGCGCTT	52	688	[25]
Endocartidis antigen (efaA)	GCCAATTGGGACAGACCCTC CGCCTTCTGTTCCTTCTTTGGC	57	688	[26]
Enterococcal surface protein (esp)	AGATTTCATCTTTGATTCTTG AATTGATTCTTTAGCATCTGG	50	510	[25]

Table 3. *Cont.*

Target Gene	Primer Sequence	Annealing Temperature (°C)	Fragment Size (bp)	Reference
Gelatinase (*gelE*)	TATGACAATGCTTTTTGGGAT AGATGCACCCGAAATAATATA	47	213	[25]
Hyluronidase (*hyl*)	ACAGAAGAGCTGCAGGAAATG GACTGACGTCCAAGTTTCCAA	53	276	[25]
Vancomycin Resistance (*vanA*)	TCTGCAATAGAGATAGCCGC GGAGTAGCTATCCCAGCATT	52	377	[26]
Vancomycin Resistance (*vanB*)	GCTCCGCAGCCTGCATGGACA ACGATGCCGCCATCCTCCTGC	60	529	[26]
Histidine decarboxylase (*hdc1*)	AGATGGTATTGTTTCTTATG AGACCATACACCATAACCTT	46	367	[27]
Histidine decarboxylase (*hdc2*)	AAYTCNTTYGAYTTYGARAARGARG ATNGGNGANCCDATCATYTTRTGNCC	50	534	[27]
Tyrosine decarboxylase (*tdc*)	GAYATNATNGGNATNGGNYTNGAYCARG CCRTARTCNGGNATAGCRAARTCNGTRTG	55	924	[27]
Ornithinedecarboxylase (*odc*)	GTNTTYAAYGCNGAYAARCANTAYTTYGT ATNGARTTNAGTTCRCAYTTYTCNGG	54	1446	[27]

2.7. Screening for Probiotics Characteristics

2.7.1. Resistance to Low pH

The survival of cultures on MRS broth buffered at four different pH values (6, 4, 3, and 2) was studied. The isolates were inoculated (1% (v/v)) in MRS broth with 4 different pH values described above and incubated at 37 °C for 48 h. Furthermore, 1ml of sample was taken at 0, 1 and 3 h of incubation and following appropriate dilutions, was inoculated into MRS agar. Finally, after the incubation at 37 °C for 48 h the forming colonies were counted. The survival ratio of the 1st and the 3rd hour was calculated using the log of the surviving cells (cfu/mL) in 1 and 3 h, divided by the log of the starting cells (cfu/mL) at 0 h [28]. The analysis was repeated three individual times.

2.7.2. Resistance to Bile Salts

Resistance to MRS broth containing 0.3% of bile acids (Sigma-Aldrich, Saint Louis, MO, USA) was tested as follows. Firstly, the samples (1% v/v)) of 0 and 3 h were received from a water bath (37 °C), following by appropriate dilutions and finally inoculated into MRS agar. Colony counting took place after 48 h of incubation at 37 °C. The survival ratio was calculated using the log of the surviving cells (cfu/mL) in 3 h divided by the log of the original cells (cfu/mL) at 0 h [29]. The analysis was repeated three individual times.

2.8. Statistical Analysis

The results were expressed as the mean and standard deviation with triplicate determinations, followed by frequencies distribution. Significant differences for microbiological and technological analyses between samples were determined using the statistical software MINITAB 12.0 by the method of one way analysis of variance (ANOVA).

Principal component analysis (PCA) was used to discriminate all isolates on the base of their technological and probiotics properties, while the discriminating variables were proteolytic activity, lipolytic activity, acidification activity, survival to pH 2 at 1 h, survival to pH 3 at 1 h, survival to pH 3 at 2 h, survival to bile salts (0.3%). Factors with eigenvalues higher than 1.00 were retained according to the Kaiser criterion [29]. In the case of not numeric values (proteolytic and lypolitic activity), before the use of PCA, it was used the method of Optimal Scaling, so our factorial points of the objects obtain new, complex, quantitative variables, which are linearly independent. PCA was performed using the statistical software SPSS v.20.

3. Results and Discussion

3.1. Microbial Enumeration

The results of total aerobic bacteria, *Enterobacteriaceae*, LAB on MRS and M17 agar, yeasts and molds, coliforms, *Micrococcaceae*, and Gram negative cocci of the fermented green cracked Cypriot table olives are summarized in Table 4. As shown in Table 4, LAB were the predominant microorganisms, having an average value of 8.04 ± 0.04 $\log_{10}$cfu/g. However, yeasts and molds counts were counted at lower levels (3.48 ± 0.06 $\log_{10}$cfu/g). In accordance with our results, in other study it was found that LAB from Spanish style fermented "Bella di Cerignola" table olives were the predominant microorganisms, having a population of 6.74 ± 0.16 $\log_{10}$cfu/g, at the end of fermentation process, while yeasts population was limited [30]. Another study reports that in natural processing of olives the predominant organisms are yeasts contrary to Lactic Acid Bacteria dominating the fermentation of Spanish style treated olives [31]. It is worthwhile to mention that in the present study, the population of *Enterobacteriaceae* and coliforms was found at quite high levels (4.66 ± 0.02 $\log_{10}$cfu/g and 3.83 ± 0.01 $\log_{10}$cfu/g, respectively), despite the low pH values (3.89 ± 0.01). *Enterobacteriaceae* can be found at the beginning of the fermentation and are quickly inhibited by pH decrease due to LAB activity which produce lactic acid as well as bacteriocins responsible of the safety of fermented products [32]. A possible justification for these high numbers of *Enterobacteriaceae* could be the short period of time (30 days) of fermentation not affecting their counts. Reports from other studies show that *Enterobacteriaceae* disappear in 30–40 days [32].

Table 4. Mean values ($\log_{10}$cfu/g; x ± SD) of the counts of different microbial groups, as well as pH values of Cypriot green cracked table olives. Mean values of three individual plate counts.

Medium	Log cfu mL^{-1}
TAC [a]	9.18 ± 0.07
Yeasts and Molds	3.48 ± 0.06
LAB on MRS agar	8.04 ± 0.04
Coliforms	4.66 ± 0.02
Enterobacteriaceae	3.83 ± 0.01
Micrococcaceae	nd *
LAB on M17 agar	4.86 ± 0.06
Salt Resistant Bacteria	7.81 ± 0.08
Gram -ve	5.37 ± 0.03
pH	3.89 ± 0.01

* nd: not detected; [a] TAC: Total Aerobic Counts.

3.2. Isolation and Identification of LAB

Ninety two colonies were randomly picked from MRS plates containing 30–300 colonies. MRS was chosen as the source of isolates because it showed the highest populations. Sixty-four Gram positive isolates were considered as LAB due to the fact that, they were cocci and catalase negative, and thus it seems that they belong to the genus of *Enterococcus*, according to the phenotypic identification (growth to all NaCl concentrations, pH and temperatures, negative to heterofermentation). Molecular identification via multiplex species specific PCR showed that all 64 isolates were *E. faecium*.

Enterococci were isolated from Spanish-style green olive fermentations [33]. Isolates have been identified, characterized, and utilized with *Lactobacillus pentosus* as starter cultures for Spanish-style green olive fermentation. In another study [10], three strains of Enterococci were isolated from olives, belonged to the species *E. faecium*. Furthermore, a total number of 52 LAB have been isolated from naturally fermented green olives collected from different areas of Sicily [11]. Even though the majority of these strains belonged to the genus of *Lactobacillus*, some of them were identified as *Enterococcus* spp., as well.

3.3. Technological Properties

3.3.1. Acidification Activity

A good mesophilic fast acid producing starter culture will reduce the pH of the milk at 5.3 after 6 h of incubation at 37 °C [24]. Of the Enterococci of the present study, none of them reduced the milk pH to <6.0 after 6 h of incubation (Figure 1, Table 5). However, after 24 h of incubation, nine out of 64 isolates reduced milk pH levels to >4.60, 34 of 64 from 5.10 to 4.60, while 21 of them kept the pH value to <5.10. Thus, those isolates could be considered as slow or medium acidifiers [34], and could be classified in three main groups: (i) those showing a high acidifying capacity, with a pH decrease of 2 pH units (14.1%) and more, (ii) those with an intermediate acidifying activity showing a pH decrease ranging from 1.5 to 2.0 pH units (53.1% of the isolates), and (iii) those with low acidifying capacity (32.8% of the isolates) showing a decrease in pH value less than 1.5 pH units (Figure 1, Table 5). It is known that the rate of acid production is a crucial factor when it comes to select a proper starter culture. Besides, pH prevents the growth of undesirable microorganisms such as spoilage and pathogenic bacteria, is also responsible for the organoleptic properties of the final product. The high capacity acidifiers (14.1%) identified, could be used as starter cultures for the production of fermented table olives because they could reduce the pH value and metabolize lactose to lactic acid. Slow or medium acidifiers (85.9%), could also be used as starter cultures in combination with the high capacity acidifiers because they have other interesting technological characteristics.

According to literature, considerable work has been done on acid production of *Enterococcus* species. In general, enterococci show low or medium acidifying ability, a fact that agrees with the present study [22]. Particularly, in another work, it has been reported that the pH value of milk did not fall below 5.5 pH units after 24 h inoculated with *E. faecium* [35]. Some other studies on enterococci confirmed the poor acidifying activity of these microorganisms in milk, giving a small percentage of strains showing a pH below 5.0–5.2 after 16–24 h of incubation at 37 °C [28,30,31]. It has been also shown that *E. faecalis* has higher acidification activity than *E. faecium* in general [36].

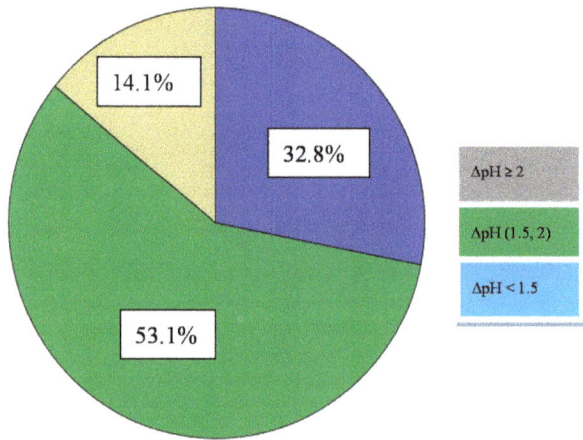

Figure 1. Percentage of number of isolates categorized in three acidification activity groups (low $\Delta pH < 1.5$, medium ΔpH (1.5, 2) and high $\Delta pH \geq 2$) after 24 h incubation at 37 °C in 10% skim milk.

Table 5. Isolates of *Enterococcus* spp. showing positive or negative proteolytic activity, positive or negative lipolytic activity, and acidification activity of high medium or low level (low ΔpH < 1.5, medium ΔpH (1.5,2) and high ΔpH ≥ 2 after 24 h incubation at 37 °C in 10% skim milk).

	Proteolytic Activity (Positives)	Proteolytic Activity (Negatives)	Lipolytic Activity (Positives)	Lipolytic Activity (Negatives)	Acidification Activity (High)	Acidification Activity (Medium)	Acidification Activity (Low)
Isolates (*Enterococcus*)	7,11–14,16–18, 27–37	1–6,8–10,15, 19–26,38–64	11–13,16–18,32, 36,42,53,54,62,63	1–10,14,15,19–31, 33,34,35,37–41, 43–52,55–61,64	3,23,26,27,28, 42,47,52,59	1,2,4–10,13,14,18, 21,22,24,25,29–33, 35,37,39,40,41,43,50, 51,55,56,57,60–64	11,12,15,16,17,19, 20,34,36,38,44, 45,46,48,49, 53,54,58

3.3.2. Proteolytic Activity

Proteolysis is one of the main industrial phenomena that contribute to the development of the organoleptic characteristics of a fermented product. The proteolytic activity of the isolates was recorded by the presence of a clear halo (positive result) on 10% Skim Milk agar. Nineteen out of 64 strains (29.7%) showed proteolytic activity. According to the literature, it has been reported that between seven strains of Enterococcus, only one was able to degrade casein, being positive for proteolytic activity [22]. Our isolates have less proteolytic activity (Figure 2a, Table 5) in comparison with other *Enterococcus* strains that have been characterized in other studies. In particular, according to other studies, enterococci were characterized having weak proteinase activity [33,36]. The same conclusion was drawn in another systematic study [34], in which 129 *E. faecium*, *E. faecalis*, and *E. durans* strains were screened for their technological characteristics. It was found that all strains showed low extracellular proteolytic activity, with the *E. faecalis* strains being more active. Generally, there are few data regarding the proteolytic system of enterococci in comparison with other LAB species. The proteolytic activity is low in *Enterococcus* strains, except of *E. faecalis* strains [30,32]. It is worthwhile to mention, that in the present study there is no correlation between proteolytic and acidification activities, because the fact that only two strains were positive to proteolytic activity, were able to reduce pH value to more than two units, as well. This finding agrees with those of a study performed by other researchers [37], suggesting that no clear relationship was observed between proteolytic and acidification activities. However, according to other report, it has been observed that the majority of the acidifying strains also had proteolytic activity [36]. Nevertheless, more and deeper physiological studies are needed in order to investigate whether or not the proteolytic ability of enterococci is one of its characteristics and how is regulated.

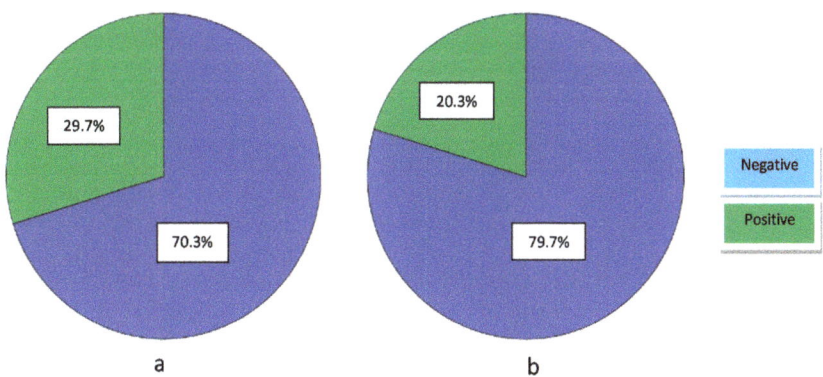

Figure 2. Percentage of number of: (**a**) proteolytic positive isolates and (**b**) lipolytic positive isolates.

3.3.3. Lipolytic Activity

The lipolytic activity is a desirable characteristic of a strain to be used as a starter culture in order to highlight certain organoleptic characteristics of the final product. Limited reports exist on the lipolytic activity of enterococci, especially those isolated from table olives. Regarding the results of this study, it seems that enterococci have generally low lipolytic activity when using tributyrin agar. Namely, only 20.31% (13 out of 64) of strains were positive to lipolytic activity (Figure 2b, Table 5). Additionally, there are some studies showing low or no lipolytic activity of *Enterococcus* species [27,31,32]. Moreover, in another work, it has been showed that the existence of lipolytic activity was only confirmed for two out of seven *Enterococcus* isolates [22]. However, there is a study reported that among 129 enterococci, the majority of them (90%) hydrolyzed all tributyrin substrates [34]. Furthermore, in the same work, it has been concluded that *E. faecalis* strains were the most lipolytic, followed by the *E. faecium* and *E. durans* strains. All studies lead to the conclusion that lipolytic activity of enterococci, is strain depended as well as related to the type of the examined food.

3.3.4. Exopolysaccharide Production (EPS)

According to our results about EPS production, all isolates were not able to produce EPS since they were showing pink to red colonies. EPS is a protection barrier against lethal influence of the environment (desiccation, phagocytosis, phage attack, osmotic stress, antibiotics or toxic compounds) and the major component of bacterial biofilm, enhancing the colonization of probiotic bacteria in cell-host interactions in the gastrointestinal tract [38]. This is a beneficial trait for probiotics in their endeavor to colonize the gut. However, according to two other studies 26 out of 72 tested strains were able to produce EPS and seven out of 25 strains, respectively [28,35]. However, more studies are required in order to learn more about the EPS production from *Enterococcus* spp.

3.3.5. β-Glucosidase Activity

None of the isolates gave positive result (blue colony), so they are not able to produce the β-glucosidase enzyme. The enzyme of β-glucosidase is closely related to the oleuropein hydrolysis and the debittering process in table olives so it is a desirable characteristic for a potential starter culture [39].

3.3.6. Catabolism of Citric Acid

Citrate metabolism by LAB is essential in a wide range of fermented foods and beverages, since it serves as a precursor for the formation of plenty other compounds contributing to the final organoleptic characteristics. None of the isolates could catabolize the citric acid as unique source of carbon. The metabolism of citric acid has been extensively studied and it is well documented in several *Lactococcus, Lactobacillus,* and *Leuconostoc* species [40]. In contrast, only a few data deals with citrate metabolism by *Enterococcus* strains are available. According to them, strains of *E. faecium* have less ability to utilize citrate as unique source of carbon [34].

3.4. Pathogenicity

Pathogenicity tests (DNase production, hemolytic activity) were negative for all strains, suggesting their safety as starter cultures but the study of virulence factors by molecular methods in *Enterococcus* spp. coming from foods, is necessary due to the risk of genetic transfer since these genes are usually located in conjugative plasmids [23,41]. The presence of virulence factors in enterococci can greatly contribute to enhance the severity of hospital infections. The isolates were tested for the presence of genes encoding potential virulence factors and biogenic amines. Five (7.8%) of our isolates were positive for *gelE* gene. However, in previous studies, it has been found that strains having this gene did not produce gelatinase [24,38], because the fsr operon could be damaged, lost, or suffer deletions due to physiological stresses from laboratory storage.. Hemolysin production increases the severity of enterococcal infections, and the presence of hemolysin/cytolysin genes is considered a risk pathogenicity factor. Regarding the *cylA* gene, two (3.1%) isolates gave a positive result, but according to phenotypical tests, only γ-hemolysis was observed. *cylA* has been considered as a "silent gene" and its gene expression can be influenced by the environmental factors and conditions used for phenotypic tests [24]. The genes *esp, efaA,* and *ace* have been involved in the colonization and adhesion at biotic and non-biotic surfaces, and the host immune system evasion. The genes *esp*, *efaA*, and *ace* were not detected in none of the isolates. However other authors found high incidence of *esp*, *asa1*, and *efaA* genes in E. faecalis [39,42]. Moreover, none of the isolates gave a positive result for *hyl*, which is related to the production of hyaluronidase facilitating the spread of toxins and bacteria throughout the host tissue by causing tissue damage. Similarly, aggregation substance (*asa1*) was not detected in our isolates. This gene is a sex pheromone plasmid-encoded surface protein, which promotes the conjugative transfer of sex pheromone plasmids by formation of mating aggregates between donor and recipient cells. Finally, none of the isolates was positive for *vanA* and *vanB* genes. This is in agreement with the results from previous studies [24,43], reporting that *vanA* and *vanB* genes have not been found frequently in enterococci isolates from food sources. However, in other work, it has been reported that three strains (50%) of *Enterococcus faecalis* were positive to *vanA* gene [22]. Regarding the presence of several-amino decarboxylase genes, histidine (*hdc1* and *hdc2*), ornithine (*odc*), and tyrosine (*tdc*) decarboxylase, no amplification occurred for either *hdc1* and *hdc2*, or *odc*. However, the *tdc* gene was present in 11 (17.1%) isolates, which is in accordance with the literature reported that despite the fact that tyramine production is a common characteristic of enterococcal isolates it is considered to be a negative trait for their possible use in foodstuffs [21,28,44].

The safety profile of enterococci isolated from Cypriot green table olive revealed that all of them were negative to the most clinically relevant antibiotics, such as *vanA* and *vanB* genes. The *van* gene is transferable, making this antibiotic resistance the most important safety factor to be evaluated in food-grade enterococci [45]. It is crucial to mention that the lack of the determinants of infectivity and antibiotic resistance in our enterococcus strains raises optimism about their further application in fermented foods. It must be mentioned that the presence of some virulence genes such like *gelE*, which was found in some of our isolates, cannot be considered as a negative trend, since enterococci are a part of the spontaneous microbiota of table olives and these genes have been also found in commercial enterococci starter cultures with a long history of safe use [44].

3.5. Screening for Probiotic Potential

Probiotic potential is one of the main factors in the case of choosing a starter culture. Tolerance to bile salts is a prerequisite for colonization and metabolic activity of probiotic bacteria in the small intestine of the host. Results indicated that all tested isolates were resistant to bile salts since the majority of them were grown successfully in MRS broth supplemented with 0.3% bile salts representing the physiological concentration of human bile (Table 6). Moreover, the isolates exhibited high tolerance to acidic conditions, surviving in pH 4.0, 5.0, and 6.0 (100% survival), in pH 2 (after 1 h of incubation), as well as in pH 3.0 (after 1 and 3 h of incubation), having high survival rates. In addition, after 3 h of incubation at pH 2.0, none of the isolates survived. However, all of isolates could be characterized as potential probiotics. According to other study among seven selected strains, three strains of *E. faecium* survived at pH 3.0 after 3 h (over 85%), while the other four strains showed lower survival rates [46]. The results indicated that all tested strains (Table 7) could possibly survive through the human stomach and might possess the ability to reach the intestinal environment in which they may effectively work. In the same work all tested strains survived in the presence of 1% bile salts over the rate 85%. Based on these results, *E. faecium* strains have the prerequisites to survive in the gastrointestinal tract. Finally, other researchers revealed that *Enterococcus* spp. strains from different sources could have the ability to reach the intestinal lumen and stay alive in that environment [28,47] However, further *in vitro* studies are needed with these strains in order to establish their probiotic potential.

Table 6. Percentage of isolates for survival at various rates to low pH and bile salts.

Survival Rate	pH 2 (1 h)	pH 3 (1 h)	pH 3 (3 h)	Bile Salts 0.3%
>70%	89%	57.8%	82.7%	10.9%
(70%, 80%)	11%	20.3%	9.5%	20.3%
(80%, 90%)	0%	12.5%	7.8%	34.4%
<90%	0%	9.4%	0%	34.4%

Table 7. Isolates of *Enterococcus* spp. surviving at different rates for various pH and exposure times or bile salts.

Survival Rate	pH 2 (1 h)	pH 3 (1 h)	pH 3 (3 h)	Bile Salts 0.3%
>70%	2–14,17,18,20, 21,22,24–64	7,8,9,10,12,13, 14,17,18,21,24,25,26, 29–39,41–46,50, 53,57,58,62,63,64	5,7,8,9,10,11,12, 13,14,17,18,20,21, 22,24–51,53,54,55,56, 57,58,59,61,62,63,64	5,7,8,17,36,37,59
(70%, 80%)	1,3,4,15,16,19,23	5,11,27,28,40,48, 49,51,54,55,56,59,61	1,2,3,4,6,16, 19,23,52,60	10,18,23,24,28,29, 35,43,45,46,52,55,58
(80%, 90%)	-	6,16,19,20,22,47,52,60	1,2,3,4,15,	9,14,15,16,20,21,22,27, 30,31,39,40,41,42,50, 51,53,54,56,57,60,61
≤90%	-	1,2,3,4,15,23	-	1,2,3,4,6,11,12,13, 19,25,26,32,33,34,38, 44,47,48,49,62,63,64

3.6. Multivariate Analysis of Phenotypic Characteristics Related to Probiotic Potential

In our study, three eigenvalues had value higher than 1. The study of the contribution of variables to factors (Table 8) showed that Factor 1 (43.19% of variance) was related to five variables (acidification activity, survival to bile salts, survival to pH 2_{1h}, survival to pH 3_{1h}, survival to pH 3_{3h}), Factor 2 (18.515% of variance) was related to one variable (lipolytic activity), and Factor 3 (13.093% of variance) to one variable (proteolytic activity) (Figure 3a). A projection of the variables on the plane formed by the first two factors (Figure 3b) shows a clear relationship between the variables described above. However, they are quite scattered among them, but they can be distinguished mainly by three groups in which are close to each other. The first group is placed on the negative part of the two factors and involves isolates that do not combine proteolysis and lipolysis (or absence of both), having low resistance to pH but quite good resistance to bile salts (up to 75%), as well. Also, the majority of them are characterized as medium acidifiers. In the second group (negative of first factor and positive of second one), they are isolates with a greater resistance to pH and bile salts than the first group, and proteolytic and lypolitic activity are combined (both presence and absence). However, in this group microorganisms are characterized as slow and/or medium acidifiers. In the third group, which is placed on the positive side of factor 1 and negative of factor 2, there are isolates with high survival to pH (more than 75% in pH 3 after 3 h) and bile salts (up to 90%). Furthermore the majority of them are high acidifiers, but they do not have proteolytic and lypolytic activity. Apart from three main groups described above, there are also a few isolates separated from the rest. For example isolates 11 and 12 have medium resistance to pH but high resistance to bile salts (93% and 100% respectively). They are also a few low acidifiers but they have both proteolytic and lipolytic activity. Furthermore, another group of four isolates (1, 2, 3, 4) was characterized by high values of acidification, while they have high resistance to pH (average 74% to pH 2 and 84% to pH 3 after 3 h) and bile salts (100%, 97% 100%, and 94%, respectively). None of these isolates have proteolytic and lipolytic activity. Isolate 16 which is depicted a bit away from the others (on positive side of factor 1 and negative of factor 2) presents intermediate values for all the parameters. According to PCA analysis, we conclude to seven isolates (1, 2, 3, 4, 11, 12, 16) having possibly promising possibly promising technological and probiotic attributes, as described above.

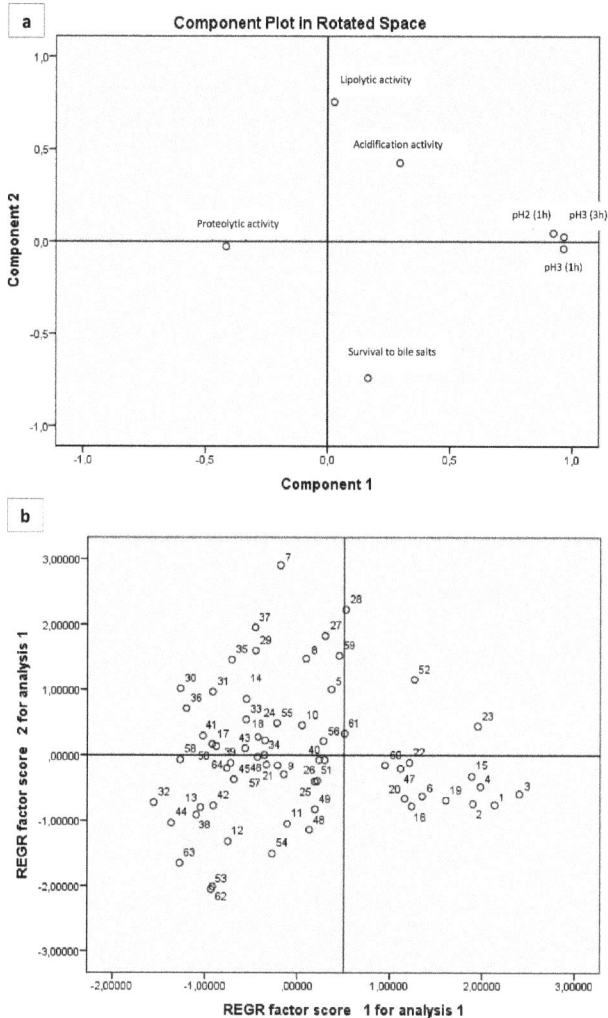

Figure 3. Projection of the variables (**a**) cases (**b**) isolates onto the plane formed by the first two factors.

Table 8. Contribution of variables (proteolytic activity, lipolytic activity, acidification activity, survival to pH 2 for 1 h, survival to pH 3 for 1 h, survival to pH 3 for 3 h and survival to bile salts) to the factors in the PCA based on correlations.

Variable	Factor 1	Factor 2	Factor 3
Proteolytic activity	−0.416	<0.01	0.683
Lipolytic activity	0.055	0.753	0.250
Acidification activity	0.311	0.413	−0.545
Survival to pH2 $_{1h}$	0.925	0.011	0.240
Survival to pH3 $_{1h}$	0.967	<0.01	0.117
Survival to pH3 $_{3h}$	0.964	<0.01	0.119
Survival to bile salts	0.139	−0.747	<0.01

4. Conclusions

This is the first comprehensive report on the characterization of LAB isolates from fermented Cypriot table olives. Enterococci were the predominant group of LAB, and it seems that those strains could find possible applications in food industry, due to their interesting technological and probiotic properties, such as their resistance to low pH and to bile salts. However, more research is required in those essential characteristics, and scientists should give more attention in the future to the genus as it becomes apparent that is a dominant group of microorganisms in fermented food products.

Author Contributions: Conceptualization, D.A.A. and D.T.; Methodology, D.A.A., D.B., D.T.; Formal Analysis, D.A.A.; Investigation, D.A.A.; Resources, D.T.; Data Curation, D.A.A., D.T.; Writing—Original Draft Preparation, D.A.A. and D.B.; Writing—Review & Editing, D.T.; Project Administration, D.T.; Funding Acquisition, D.T.

Funding: This study was funded by internal funds from the Cyprus University of Technology to Dimitris Tsaltas.

Acknowledgments: The authors gratefully acknowledge the material provided by A. Agathokleous (King of Olives, Agglissides, Larnaca, Cyprus) and the financial support from the Cyprus University of Technology to Dimitris Tsaltas.

Conflicts of Interest: The authors declare no conflict of interest.

References

1. Olives, T. *No 66—November 2012*; International Olive Council: Madrid, Spain, 2012.
2. López, F.N.A.; Romero, C.; Quintana, M.D.C.D.; López, A.L.; García, P.G.; Fernández, A.G. Kinetic study of the physicochemical and microbiological changes in 'seasoned' olives during the shelf-life period. *J. Agric. Food Chem.* **2005**, *53*, 5285–5292. [CrossRef] [PubMed]
3. Bautista-Gallego, J.; Arroyo-López, F.N.; Rantsiou, K.; Jiménez-Díaz, R.; Garrido-Fernández, A.; Cocolin, L. Screening of lactic acid bacteria isolated from fermented table olives with probiotic potential. *Food Res. Int.* **2013**, *50*, 135–142. [CrossRef]
4. Montet, D.; Ray, R.C.; Zakhia-Rozis, N. Lactic Acid Fermentation of Vegetables and Fruits. In *Microorganisms and Fermentation of Traditional Foods*; CRC Press: Boca Raton, FL, USA, 2014; pp. 108–140.
5. Stiles, M.E.; Holzapfel, W.H. Lactic acid bacteria of foods and their current taxonomy. *Int. J. Food Microbiol.* **1997**, *36*, 1–29. [CrossRef]
6. Fisher, K.; Phillips, C. The ecology, epidemiology and virulence of *Enterococcus*. *Microbiology* **2009**, *155*, 1749–1757. [CrossRef] [PubMed]
7. Lebreton, F.; Willems, R.J.L.; Gilmore, M.S. Enterococcus Diversity, Origins in Nature, and Gut Colonization. In *Enterococci: From Commensals to Lead. Causes Drug Resistant Infection*; Massachusetts Eye and Ear Infirmary: Boston, MA, USA, 2014; pp. 1–56.
8. Franz, C.M.A.P.; Huch, M.; Abriouel, H.; Holzapfel, W.; Gálvez, A. Enterococci as probiotics and their implications in food safety. *Int. J. Food Microbiol.* **2011**, *151*, 125–140. [CrossRef] [PubMed]
9. Gomes, B.C.; Dora, B.; de Melo, G.; De Martinis, E.C.P.; Paulo, S. Dualistic aspects of *Enterococcus* spp. in foods. *Curr. Res. Technol. Educ. Top. Appl. Microbiol. Microb. Biotechnol.* **2010**, 1119–1125.
10. Omar, N.B.; Castro, A.; Lucas, R.; Abriouel, H.; Yousif, N.M.K.; Franz, C.M.A.P.; Holzapfel, W.H.; Ruben, P.P.; Martínez-Cañamero, M.; Gálvez, A. Functional and Safety Aspects of Enterococci Isolated from Different Spanish Foods. *Syst. Appl. Microbiol.* **2004**, *27*, 118–130. [CrossRef] [PubMed]
11. Randazzo, C.L.; Restuccia, C.; Romano, A.D.; Caggia, C. *Lactobacillus casei*, dominant species in naturally fermented Sicilian green olives. *Int. J. Food Microbiol.* **2004**, *90*, 9–14. [CrossRef]
12. Gonza, J.M.; Lucena-padro, H.; Ruiz-barba, L.; Maldonado-Barraga, A. *Enterococcus olivae* sp. nov., isolated from Spanish-style green-olive fermentations. *Int. J. Syst. Evol. Microbiol.* **2014**, *64*, 2534–2539.
13. Shinozaki-Kuwahara, N.; Saito, M.; Hirasawa, M.; Hirasawa, M.; Takada, K. *Streptococcus dentiloxodontae* sp. nov., isolated from the oral cavity of elephants. *Int. J. Syst. Evol. Microbiol.* **2016**, *66*, 3878–3883. [PubMed]
14. Cogan, T.M. Characterization of the lactic acid bacteria in artisanal dairy products. *J. Dairy Res.* **1997**, *64*, 409–421. [CrossRef]
15. Estifanos, H. Isolation and identification of probiotic lactic acid bacteria from curd and in vitro evaluation of its growth inhibition activities against pathogenic bacteria. *Afr. J. Microbiol. Res.* **2014**, *8*, 1419–1425. [CrossRef]

16. Jackson, C.R.; Fedorka-Cray, P.J.; Barrett, J.B. Use of a Genus- and Species-Specific Multiplex PCR for Identification of Enterococci Use of a Genus- and Species-Specific Multiplex PCR for Identification of Enterococci. *J. Clin. Microbiol.* **2004**, *42*, 3558. [CrossRef] [PubMed]
17. Fuka, M.M.; Maksimovic, A.Z.; Tanuwidjaja, I.; Hulak, N.; Schloter, M. Characterization of enterococcal community isolated from an Artisan Istrian raw milk cheese: Biotechnological and safety aspects. *Food Technol. Biotechnol.* **2017**, *55*, 368–380.
18. Franciosi, E.; Settanni, L.; Cavazza, A.; Poznanski, E. Biodiversity and technological potential of wild lactic acid bacteria from raw cows' milk. *Int. Dairy J.* **2009**, *19*, 3–11. [CrossRef]
19. Dinçer, E.; Kıvanç, M. Lipolytic Activity of Lactic Acid Bacteria Isolated from Turkish Pastırma. *Anadolu Univ. J. Sci. Technol. C Life Sci. Biotechnol.* **2018**, *7*, 12–19. [CrossRef]
20. Imène, K.; Halima, Z.-K.; Nour-Eddine, K. Screening of exopolysaccharide-producing coccal lactic acid bacteria isolated from camel milk and red meat of Algeria. *Afr. J. Biotechnol.* **2017**, *16*, 1078–1084. [CrossRef]
21. Ghabbour, N.; Lamzira, Z.; Thonart, P.; Cidalia, P.; Markaoui, M.; Asehraou, A. Selection of oleuropein-degrading lactic acid bacteria strains isolated from fermenting Moroccan green olives. *Grasas Aceites* **2011**, *62*, 84–89.
22. Ribeiro, S.C.; Coelho, M.C.; Todorov, S.D.; Franco, B.D.G.M.; Dapkevicius, M.L.E.; Silva, C.C.G. Technological properties of bacteriocin-producing lactic acid bacteria isolated from Pico cheese an artisanal cow's milk cheese. *J. Appl. Microbiol.* **2014**, *116*, 573–585. [CrossRef] [PubMed]
23. Chajęcka-Wierzchowska, W.; Zadernowska, A.; Łaniewska-Trokenheim, Ł. Virulence factors of *Enterococcus* spp. presented in food. *LWT Food Sci. Technol.* **2017**, *75*, 670–676. [CrossRef]
24. Aspri, M.; Bozoudi, D.; Tsaltas, D.; Hill, C.; Papademas, P. Raw donkey milk as a source of *Enterococcus* diversity: Assessment of their technological properties and safety characteristics. *Food Control* **2017**, *73*, 81–90. [CrossRef]
25. Vankerckhoven, V.; van Autgaerden, T.; Vael, C.; Lammens, C.; Chapelle, S.; Rossi, R.; Jabes, D.; Goossens, H. Development of a multiplex PCR for the detection of asaI, gelE, cylA, esp, and hyl genes in enterococci and survey for virulence determinants among european hospital isolates of *Enterococcus faecium*. *J. Clin. Microbiol.* **2004**, *42*, 4473–4479. [CrossRef] [PubMed]
26. Martín-Platero, A.M.; Valdivia, E.; Maqueda, M.; Martínez-Bueno, M. Characterization and safety evaluation of enterococci isolated from Spanish goats' milk cheeses. *Int. J. Food Microbiol.* **2009**, *132*, 24–32. [CrossRef] [PubMed]
27. De las Rivas, B.; Marcobal, Á.; Muñoz, R. Improved multiplex-PCR method for the simultaneous detection of food bacteria producing biogenic amines. *FEMS Microbiol. Lett.* **2005**, *244*, 367–372. [CrossRef] [PubMed]
28. Ilavenil, S.; Park, H.S.; Vijayakumar, M.; Arasu, M.V.; Kim, D.H.; Ravikumar, S.; Choi, K.C. Probiotic Potential of *Lactobacillus* Strains with Antifungal Activity Isolated from Animal Manure. *Sci. World J.* **2015**, *2015*, 802570. [CrossRef] [PubMed]
29. Song, M.; Yun, B.; Moon, J.-H.; Park, D.-J.; Lim, K.; Oh, S. Characterization of Selected *Lactobacillus* Strains for Use as Probiotics. *Korean J. Food Sci. Anim. Resour.* **2015**, *35*, 551–556. [CrossRef] [PubMed]
30. Campaniello, D.; Bevilacqua, A.; D'Amato, D.; Corbo, M.R.; Altieri, C.; Sinigaglia, M. Microbial characterization of table olives processed according to Spanish and natural styles. *Food Technol. Biotechnol.* **2005**, *43*, 289–294.
31. Aponte, M.; Ventorino, V.; Blaiotta, G.; Volpe, G.; Farina, V.; Avellone, G.; Lanza, C.M.; Moschetti, G. Study of green Sicilian table olive fermentations through microbiological, chemical and sensory analyses. *Food Microbiol.* **2010**, *27*, 162–170. [CrossRef] [PubMed]
32. Panagou, E.Z.; Tassou, C.C.; Katsaboxakis, C.Z. Induced lactic acid fermentation of untreated green olives of the Conservolea cultivar by *Lactobacillus pentosus*. *J. Sci. Food Agric.* **2003**, *83*, 667–674. [CrossRef]
33. De Castro, A.; Montano, A.; Casado, F.-J.; Sanchez, A.-H.; Rejano, L. Utilization of Enterococcus casseliflavus and Lactobacillus pentosus as starter cultures for Spanish-style green olive fermentation. *Food Microbiol.* **2002**, *19*, 637–644. [CrossRef]
34. Sarantinopoulos, P.; Andrighetto, C.; Georgalaki, M.D.; Rea, M.C.; Lombardi, A.; Cogan, T.M.; Kalantzopoulos, G.; Tsakalidou, E. Biochemical properties of enterococci relevant to their technological performance. *Int. Dairy J.* **2001**, *11*, 621–647. [CrossRef]

35. Morea, M.; Baruzzi, F.; Cocconcelli, P.S. Molecular and physiological characterization of dominant bacterial populations in traditional Mozzarella cheese processing. *J. Appl. Microbiol.* **1999**, *87*, 574–582. [CrossRef] [PubMed]
36. Suzzi, G.; Caruso, M.; Gardini, F.; Lombardi, A.; Vannini, L.; Guerzoni, M.E.; Andrighetto, C.; Lanorte, M.T. A survey of the enterococci isolated from an artisanal Italian goat's cheese (semicotto caprino). *J. Appl. Microbiol.* **2000**, *89*, 267–274. [CrossRef] [PubMed]
37. Durlu özkaya, F.; Xanthopoulos, V.; Tunail, N.; Litopoulou-Tzanetaki, E. Technologically important properties of lactic acid bacteria isolates from Beyaz cheese made from raw ewes' milk. *J. Appl. Microbiol.* **2001**, *91*, 861–870. [CrossRef] [PubMed]
38. Kanmani, P.; Suganya, K.; Kumar, R.S.; Yuvaraj, N.; Pattukumar, V.; Paari, K.A.; Arul, V. Synthesis and functional characterization of antibiofilm exopolysaccharide produced by *Enterococcus faecium* mc13 isolated from the gut of fish. *Appl. Biochem. Biotechnol.* **2013**, *169*, 1001–1015. [CrossRef] [PubMed]
39. Charoenprasert, S.; Mitchell, A. Factors influencing phenolic compounds in table olives (*Olea europaea*). *J. Agric. Food Chem.* **2012**, *60*, 7081–7095. [CrossRef] [PubMed]
40. Laëtitia, G.; Pascal, D.; Yann, D. The Citrate Metabolism in Homo- and Heterofermentative LAB: A Selective Means of Becoming Dominant over Other Microorganisms in Complex Ecosystems. *Food Nutr. Sci.* **2014**, *5*, 953–969. [CrossRef]
41. González, L.; Sacristán, N.; Arenas, R.; Fresno, J.M.; Tornadijo, M.E. Enzymatic activity of lactic acid bacteria (with antimicrobial properties) isolated from a traditional Spanish cheese. *Food Microbiol.* **2010**, *27*, 592–597. [CrossRef] [PubMed]
42. Creti, R.; Imperi, M.; Bertuccini, L.; Fabretti, F.; Orefici, G.; Rosa, R.D.; Baldassarri, L. Survey for virulence determinants among *Enterococcus faecalis* isolated from different sources. *J. Med. Microbiol.* **2004**, *53*, 13–20. [CrossRef] [PubMed]
43. Franz, C.; Muscholl-Silberhorn, A.; Yousif, N.; Vancanneyt, M.; Swings, J.; Holzapfel, W. Incidence of virulence factors and antibiotic resistance among enterococci isolated from food. *Appl. Environ. Microbiol.* **2001**, *67*, 4385–4389. [CrossRef] [PubMed]
44. Rosado, D.; Brito, J.C.; Harris, D.J. Molecular screening of *Hepatozoon* (Apicomplexa: Adeleorina) infections in *Python sebae* from West Africa using 18S rRNA gene sequences. *Herpetol. Notes* **2015**, *8*, 461–463.
45. Klein, G. Taxonomy, ecology and antibiotic resistance of enterococci from food and the gastro-intestinal tract. *Int. J. Food Microbiol.* **2003**, *88*, 123–131. [CrossRef]
46. Strompfová, V.; Lauková, A.; Ouwehand, A.C. Selection of enterococci for potential canine probiotic additives. *Vet. Microbiol.* **2004**, *100*, 107–114. [CrossRef] [PubMed]
47. Martin, B.; Garriga, M.; Hugas, M.; Aymerich, T. Genetic diversity and safety aspects of enterococci from slightly fermented sausages. *J. Appl. Microbiol.* **2005**, *98*, 1177–1190. [CrossRef] [PubMed]

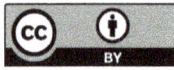 © 2018 by the authors. Licensee MDPI, Basel, Switzerland. This article is an open access article distributed under the terms and conditions of the Creative Commons Attribution (CC BY) license (http://creativecommons.org/licenses/by/4.0/).

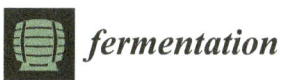

Article

Principal Component Analysis for Clustering Probiotic-Fortified Beverage Matrices Efficient in Elimination of *Shigella* sp.

Srijita Sireswar [1], Didier Montet [2] and Gargi Dey [1,*]

[1] School of Biotechnology, Kalinga Institute of Industrial Technology, Patia, Bhubaneswar, Odisha 751024, India; sireswar.srijita@gmail.com
[2] UMR Qualisud, CIRAD, TAB-95/16 73, rue Jean-François, Breton 34398, France; didier.montet@cirad.fr
* Correspondence: drgargi.dey@gmail.com; Tel.: +91-674-272-5466

Received: 19 April 2018; Accepted: 3 May 2018; Published: 8 May 2018

Abstract: Vast amounts of information can be obtained by systematic explorations of synergy between phytochemicals and probiotics, which is required for the development of non-dairy probiotic products, globally. Evidence confirms that the same probiotic strain can have different efficiencies depending on the food matrix. One such functional property, viz., antipathogenicity of the probiotic strain against *Shigella* was investigated in this study. The potential of two fruit based (apple and sea buckthorn) beverage matrices fortified with *Lactobacillus rhamnosus* GG (ATCC 53103), against outbreak-causing serotypes of *Shigella dysenteriae* (ATCC 29026) and *Shigella flexneri* (ATCC 12022) was evaluated. The originality of this study lies in the fact that the functionality assessment was performed with a more realistic approach under storage conditions from 0–14 days at 4 °C. The finding confirms that *Lactobacillus rhamnosus* GG (LGG) differs in its potential depending on beverage matrices. Principal Component Analysis (PCA) clustered the matrices based on their pathogen clearance. LGG fortified sea buckthorn beverage matrix showed 99% clearance of *S. dysenteriae* within the first hour compared to 11% in apple beverage matrix. Interestingly, *S. flexneri* showed more resistance and was cleared (99%) in the LGG fortified sea buckthorn beverage matrix within three hours compared to 5.6% in apple matrix.

Keywords: PCA; *L. rhamnosus* GG; sea buckthorn; *Shigella*

---

1. Introduction

Infectious diarrhea is one of the leading causes of mortality in developing and under developed countries [1]. In 2015, approximately 2.3 billion illnesses and 1.3 million deaths were reported due to diarrheal diseases worldwide, out of which children below five years of age accounted for 40% of diarrheal deaths [2]. The major bacterial entero-pathogens reported as etiological agents for diarrhea associated diseases are *Shigella*, entero-toxigenic *E. coli*, *Salmonella*, *Yersenia* and *Campylobacter* [3]. Shigellosis—a severe foodborne illness caused by *Shigella*—is an invasive infection of the colon, characterized by a series of systemic manifestations, beginning from short-lasting diarrhea to acute inflammatory bowel disease [4]. *Shigella* sp. is highly communicable at an extremely low infectivity dose, and is generally transmitted person-to-person as a result of poor hygiene [5]. Shigellosis results in about 800,000 fatalities annually throughout the world, predominantly in Sub-Saharan Africa and South Asia [6,7]. The Global Enteric Multicenter Study (GEMS) on the burden and etiology of moderate-to-severe diarrheal illness (MSD) established *Shigella* as 1 of 4 top pathogens in Sub-Saharan Africa and South-East Asia [8]. Among South-East Asian countries, the occurrence rate of Shigellosis was highest in India (21.7%), followed by Cambodia (19.8%), Philippines (17.9%), and Vietnam (9.0%) [9]. While antimicrobial agents are the mainstay of therapy, the emergence of drug resistance has limited the choice of antibiotics for treating Shigellosis [4,10]. Additionally, the negative influences of antibiotics on gut-microbiota homeostasis have paved the way for alternative treatments of Shigellosis [11].

Probiotics are an efficient alternative therapy for acute infectious gastroenteritis and diarrhea-associated diseases [12]. This is mainly due to immune stimulation and immunomodulatory effects, together with the modulation of the gut microflora [13]. Several studies have reported the beneficial effect of probiotics against entero-pathogenic infections [14,15]. Zhang et al. (2011) reported strong antimicrobial action of four probiotic strains, *Lactobacillus paracasei* subp. *paracasei* M5-L, *Lactobacillus rhamnosus* J10-L, *Lactobacillus casei* Q8-L and *L. rhamnosus* GG (LGG) against *Shigella* sp. [16]. Similarly, Kakisu et al. (2013) explained the antagonistic potential of *L. plantarum* CIDCA 83114, against *Shigella flexneri* and *Shigella soneii* [17].

Evidence from these observations have paved the way for probiotic functional foods [18,19]. Various foods and beverages have been explored as second-generation vehicles for probiotic delivery [20–22]. One such class of vehicles are fruits and vegetable matrices [23,24]. However, selection of an appropriate food system as a delivery matrix remains a crucial factor, since the finished products need to have adequate probiotic viability, acceptable sensory attributes and potent bio-efficacies [25–27]. There exists a two-way relationship between plant phenolics and gut microflora [28]. Gut microflora, including probiotics, are mostly anaerobes or facultative aerobes; therefore, these phenolic compounds are acting as antioxidants that scavenge and reduce the oxygen, thereby promoting its growth [29]. Furthermore, phenolic compounds enhance the potential of probiotics to produce antimicrobial compounds, thereby upgrading the safety of food and human health [30].

Earlier we have explored two phenolic-rich beverage matrices—apple (APJ) and sea buckthorn (SBT) based matrices—as probiotic delivery vehicles. We demonstrated efficacious pathogen clearance of entero-pathogenic *E. coli* (ATCC 43887), *Salmonella enteritidis* (ATCC 13076), *Shigella dysenteriae* (ATCC 29026) and non-pathogenic *E. coli* (ATCC 25922) in freshly made beverage matrices [31,32]. However, in order to be effective, any probiotic fortified beverage must retain effectiveness of the probiotic strain in spite of a long shelf life. In this study, we have applied principal component analysis (PCA) to cluster the response of different beverage matrices based on their anti-*Shigella* potential, when stored for 14 days at 4 °C.

2. Materials and Methods

2.1. Raw Materials and Bacterial Strains

Malt extract powder (M) (Imperial Malts Ltd., Gurgaon, Haryana, India), was the major ingredient used to prepare the probiotic fortified apple and sea buckthorn beverages. Probiotic Lactic Acid Bacteria (LAB), *Lactobacillus rhamnosus* GG (ATCC 53103) was used for the fortification in the fruit matrices. Pathogenic strains of *Shigella*, namely, *Shigella dysenteriae* (ATCC 29026), and *Shigella flexneri* (ATCC 12022) were used as test organisms in this study. All strains were procured from American Type Culture Collection (Microbiologics, MN, USA).

2.2. Development of Juice Matrices

The fruit based probiotic beverages were prepared according to Sireswar et al. (2017) [31]. Briefly, fresh apples and sea buckthorn berries were collected from Himachal Pradesh, India and were subjected to juice extraction, filtration and adjusted to pH 4.5 with tri-sodium citrate (Sigma-Aldrich Co., St Louis, MO, USA). The freshly extracted sea buckthorn and apple juice were separately supplemented with M at a concentration of 5% (w/v) and pasteurized at 95 °C for 5 min. The 2 juice matrices, namely, M-supplemented apple juice (APJ + M) and M-supplemented sea buckthorn juice (SBT + M) were individually fortified with approximately 8 log cfu/mL of *L. rhamnosus* GG (ATCC 53103) (LR), namely, *L. rhamnosus* GG fortified, malt-supplemented apple juice (APJ + M + LR) and *L. rhamnosus* GG fortified, malt-supplemented sea buckthorn juice (SBT + M + LR). All probiotic beverages were tightly sealed and stored at 4 °C for further evaluation.

2.3. Evaluation of Anti-Shigella Potential of the Probiotic Beverages during Shelf Storage

The anti-*Shigella* potential of the probiotic beverages were evaluated according to Sireswar et al. (2017) with slight modifications [31]. A known volume of each probiotic-fortified beverage (containing approximately 8 log cfu/mL of probiotic), were inoculated with about 6 log cfu/mL of each strain, *Shigella dysenteriae* and *Shigella flexneri*, and incubated at 37 °C for 48 h. Aliquots of the sample were taken at 0, 1, 2, 3, 4, 8, 24 and 48 h to enumerate both the pathogens as well as the probiotics. At each time interval, the sample was serially diluted and plated on MacConkey agar for pathogens and incubated at 37 °C for 24 h, and on MRS agar plates for probiotics were incubated at 37 °C for 48 h. The same procedure was repeated at equal intervals up to 14 days of shelf storage at 4 °C. The data are expressed in terms of percentage pathogen clearance:

$$\text{log reduction (L)} = \log_{10} A - \log_{10} B \qquad (1)$$

where A is the initial cfu/mL and B is the final cfu/mL of the pathogen. The initial and final log cfu data has been mentioned in Tables S1 and S2 in the Supplementary File.

$$\text{percentage pathogen clearance (\%)} = (1 - 10^{-L}) \times 100 \qquad (2)$$

2.4. Total Phenolic Content (TPC)

The total phenolic content of the probiotic beverages (APJ + M + LR and SBT + M + LR) were analyzed according to the Folin–Ciocalteu method by Singleton et al. (1999) [33]. Briefly, 20 µL of each juice sample was added to 1.58 mL of water and 100 µL of Folin–Ciocalteu reagent (Sigma-Aldrich co.). The mixture was vortexed for 30 s and allowed to stand for 5 min. To the mixture, 300 µL of saturated sodium carbonate was added and incubated at 20 °C for 2 h and absorbance was determined at 765 nm. The results were expressed as µg/mL of Gallic Acid Equivalent (GAE) using a Gallic acid standard curve of 0, 50, 100, 150, 250 and 500 µg GAE/mL. Unfortified juice matrices were taken as control (APJ + M and SBT + M).

2.5. Statistical Analysis

To test the significance of the antagonistic potential of each beverage against the *Shigella* strains, Principal Component Analysis (PCA) was applied to the percentage pathogen clearance data set through multivariate exploratory techniques using XLSTAT software (version 2015.6, Addinsoft, SARL, Paris, France). A data matrix was constructed where the samples from each interval, that is 0, 7 and 14 days, were inserted in rows and the antagonistic potential against each strain at each hour of co-incubation were placed in columns and 2D plots were generated to predict the variability among the principal components. All total phenolic content (TPC) data are as an average of triplicate experiments with standard deviation.

3. Results and Discussion

Percentage Pathogen Clearance and Principal Component Analysis (PCA)

It is well known that plant phenolic compounds have a significant impact on the functionality of probiotics [34–36]. A few reports specifically on the potential of sea buckthorn and apple juice against *Shigella* sp. also exist [37,38]. The complex matrix environment and its physicochemical attributes, especially of beverage matrices for probiotic delivery, alter the potential of probiotic strains by modifying their efficacy and functionality during storage [39]. There is sufficient evidence of change in functionality of probiotics without any alteration in the level of viable cells during storage [40].

Hence, it is necessary to know the alterations that may occur in the functionality of probiotics in a food matrix during storage, even though the viable count may not have changed. Earlier we have reported the symbiosis of apple and sea buckthorn phenolics, with probiotic action against entero-pathogens [31]. Those observations formed the premise for the current evaluation, where we apply PCA to evaluate the efficiency of the influence of beverage matrices fortified with *L. rhamnosus* GG for elimination of *Shigella dysenteriae* and *Shigella flexneri* during a storage period.

Tables 1 and 2 represent the percentage pathogen clearance of the unfortified matrices, APJ + M, SBT + M, and probiotic fortified beverages, APJ + M + LR and SBT + M + LR during shelf storage at regular intervals (Day 0, Day 7 and Day 14) against *S. dysenteriae* and *S. flexneri*, respectively. Results indicated that the highest pathogen clearance was demonstrated in SBT + M + LR against both *Shigella* species. A pathogen clearance of 99.99% was observed within 1 h of co-incubation in SBT + M + LR at day 0 against *S. dysenteriae*. Similar pathogen clearance (99.99%) was observed only after 4 h in APJ + M + LR. For SBT + M + LR, when co-incubated for 1 h with *S. flexneri*, only 8.4% clearance was shown, and for APJ + M + LR clearance was as low as 5.09%. However, *S. flexneri* was finally eliminated after 3 h of incubation in the case of SBT + M + LR. Interestingly, SBT + M + LR, when stored for 7 days showed nearly complete pathogen clearance after a lag of 2 h, and APJ + M + LR after lag of 4 h, indicating that storage may influence the functionality of the probiotic. Similar functional evaluations of stored probiotic beverages fortified with LGG have not been carried out and hence are not available for comparison. However, a somewhat similar assessment of elimination of *P. aeruginosa*, *E. coli*, *S. aureus* and *S. enteritidis* by *L. casei* and *B. animalis*-fortified whey cheese matrix was performed by Madureira et al. (2011) [40]. The authors reported elimination of *E. coli*, *S. aureus* and *S. enteritidis* at the much lower contaminant inoculum level of 10^3–10^4 cfu/g after a much longer co-incubation period. No elimination was observed with respect to *P. aeruginosa* in *L. casei*-fortified matrix after 14 days of storage [40].

Another important observation of the study was that fortification of probiotic strain *L. rhamnosus* GG significantly enhanced the anti-*Shigella* potential of both SBT and APJ matrices. Unfortified juice matrices (SBT + M) showed 76.1% pathogen clearance for *S. dysenteriae* and 56% pathogen clearance for *S. flexneri* after 8 h of co-incubation. While comparing the two pathogens, *S. dysenteriae* was more easily susceptible to inhibition than *S. flexneri*. This may be because of the higher stress resistance and acid tolerance of *S. flexneri*. In and colleagues in 2013 reported the sensitivity of *S. dysenteriae* to organic acids in comparison to other *Shigella* serotypes, namely, *S. soneii*, *S. boydii* and *S. flexneri* [41]. Our results corroborate the previous results of Bagamboula et al. (2002), which established the survival of *S. flexneri* in highly acidic apple juice for 14 days [42]. The lag in pathogen inhibition could also be due to the hfq protein in *S. flexneri*, acting as a key factor in maximal adaptation to environmental stress—especially low pH conditions—thereby regulating acid stress tolerance within the matrix environment [43].

Table 1. Percentage pathogen clearance potential of *L. rhamnosus* GG fortified sea buckthorn (SBT) and apple juice (APJ) against *Shigella dysteneriae* during 14 days of shelf storage.

Percentage Pathogen Clearance (%)	1 h	2 h	3 h	4 h	8 h
SBT + M (Day 0)	6.78	9.88	17.26	37.82	76.1
SBT + M (Day 7)	5.56	8.19	27.92	48.19	69.37
SBT + M (Day 14)	4.48	9.16	11.28	28.28	69.29
SBT + M + LR (Day 0)	99.99	99.99	99.99	99.99	99.99
SBT + M + LR (Day 7)	99.26	99.62	99.99	99.99	99.99
SBT + M + LR (Day 14)	89.28	99.08	99.99	99.99	99.99
APJ + M (Day 0)	5.43	8.12	10.75	20.18	57.19
APJ + M (Day 7)	4.49	8	11.18	26.27	52.16
APJ + M (Day 14)	4.41	7.72	16.9	22.27	55.34
APJ + M + LR (Day 0)	10.75	15.28	91.68	99.99	99.99
APJ + M + LR (Day 7)	9.26	10.26	13.43	92.89	99.99
APJ + M + LR (Day 14)	8.27	9.17	15.29	90.48	99.99

Table 2. Percentage pathogen clearance potential of *L. rhamnosus* GG fortified sea buckthorn (SBT) and apple juice (APJ) against *Shigella flexneri* during 14 days of shelf storage.

Percentage Pathogen Clearance (%)	1 h	2 h	3 h	4 h	8 h
SBT + M (Day 0)	4.7	5.67	10.18	22.19	56.1
SBT + M (Day 7)	4.56	6.18	17.98	27.63	54.29
SBT + M (Day 14)	4.3	5.56	6.11	28.82	55.28
SBT + M + LR (Day 0)	8.4	90.58	99.73	99.87	99.99
SBT + M + LR (Day 7)	8.38	17.19	90.3	99.36	99.99
SBT + M + LR (Day 14)	8.29	11.19	90.26	99.17	99.99
APJ + M (Day 0)	4.67	4.89	5.08	5.78	42.98
APJ + M (Day 7)	4.3	6.19	8.19	28.98	40.17
APJ + M (Day 14)	4.29	5.56	6.98	30.27	40.1
APJ + M + LR (Day 0)	5.09	5.18	5.56	6.87	99.99
APJ +M + LR (Day 7)	4.08	5.09	5.42	5.95	90.72
APJ + M + LR (Day 14)	4	5.18	5.87	6.9	90.36

To distinctively discriminate the pathogen clearance ability of the probiotic fortified matrices, we carried out a Principal Component Analysis (PCA) based on their anti-Shigella potential during shelf storage. This analysis is of importance as it provides an indication of the matrix-specific pathogen clearance potential. The biplot (Figure 1) explains 96.31% of total variation, with factor 1 on x-axis depicting 80.49% of the data and factor 2 on the y-axis explaining 15.83%. Similarly, in Figure 2, the biplot explains 89.57% of total variation, with factor 1 on x-axis depicting 76.84% of the data and factor 2 on the y-axis explaining 12.73%. Factor 1 accounts for the highest percentage pathogen clearance against *S. dysenteriae* and *S. flexneri* respectively. Factor 2 was characterized by the lag in time with respect to pathogen clearance.

The PCA biplot (Figures 1 and 2) illustrated specific functionality differences between matrices and clustered the beverages according to their composition; Cluster I—SBT + M + LR, Cluster II—APJ + M + LR, Cluster III—APJ + M and SBT + M. As mentioned earlier, the absence of probiotics had a negative impact on the pathogen clearance ability of the juice matrices.

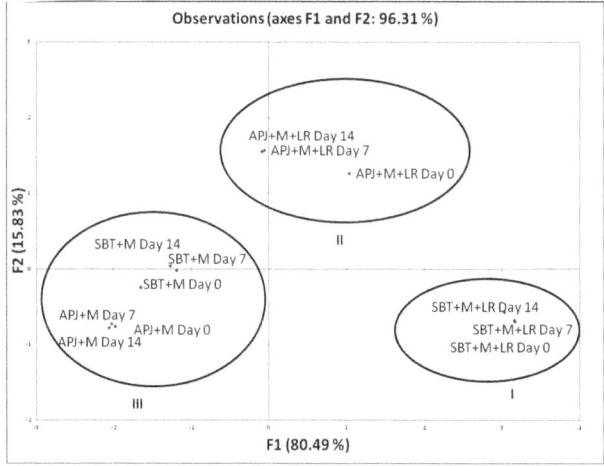

Figure 1. PCA biplot of the percentage pathogen clearance of unfortified matrices and *L. rhamnosus* GG fortified beverages against *S. dysenteriae*. The anti-*S. dysenteriae* activity of the LGG fortified beverages were performed at regular intervals (Day 0, Day 7 and Day 14) during the storage period. *S. dysenteriae* was co-incubated in different beverage matrices at 37 °C and evaluated for viable counts. The pathogen clearance percentage was calculated as per the formula provided in Section 2.3.

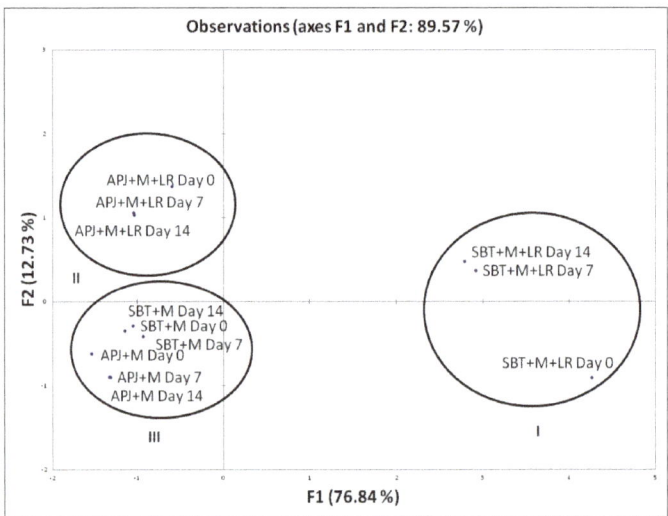

Figure 2. PCA biplot of the percentage pathogen clearance of unfortified matrices and *L. rhamnosus* GG fortified beverages against *S. flexneri*. The anti-*S. flexneri* activity of the LGG fortified beverages were performed at regular intervals (Day 0, Day 7 and Day 14) during the storage period. *S. dysenteriae* was co-incubated in different beverage matrices at 37 °C and evaluated for viable counts. The pathogen clearance percentage was calculated as per the formula provided in Section 2.3.

Another important conclusion that may be drawn from the PCA is that among probiotic fortified beverages, the total phenolic content of the matrices also influenced the efficiency. A synergistic interaction of probiotics along with phenolics is indicated. Reports of the selective stimulation of probiotic strains *Lactobacillus bulgaricus* and *Bifidibacterium bifidis* in pasteurized blueberry juice along with the inhibition of several foodborne pathogens indicated that irrespective of the presence of a probiotic strain, the phenolic content synergistically played a role in the elimination of both the Shigella stains [44]. To confirm the synergistic role, the total phenolic content of the beverage matrices were estimated (Figure 3). The SBT + M + LR had nearly two-fold more phenolic content (663.18 µgGAE/mL) as compared to APJ + M + LR (342.87 µgGAE/mL).

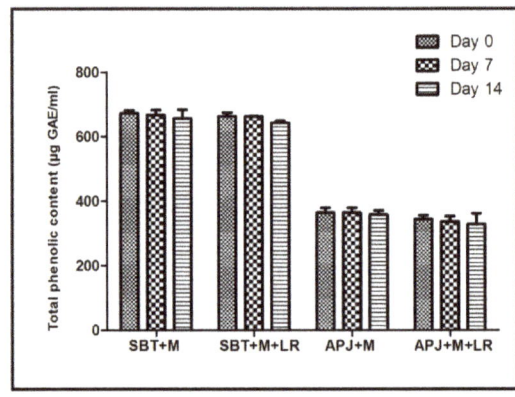

Figure 3. Total phenolic content of unfortified and *L. rhamnosus* GG fortified sea buckthorn and apple beverages during 14 days of cold storage.

Importantly, under storage conditions, the levels of phenolics in the beverage matrices did not change significantly during the 14 days period. Thus, it may be concluded that the functionality difference and the clustering shown by the beverage matrices is due to the two differentiators, viz., the presence of probiotics and presence of phenolics. In future we will be reporting on the phenolic profile of the matrices.

Some articles have been dedicated to the evaluation of antipathogenic potential of dairy probiotic products [45–47]. This is probably a rare study where the probiotic functionality has been evaluated in fruit beverage matrix with respect to its antipathogenic activity in more realistic conditions where it has been stored for 7–14 days at 4 °C.

4. Conclusions

We were able to successfully establish that together, phenolic and probiotic strain, *L. rhamnosus* GG can form an effective barrier against two potent diarrhea-causing *Shigella* strains. Such rational designing of fruit based probiotic beverages could be of great help to second-generation probiotic product developers who could utilize competitive LAB strains and juice phenolics for creating effective barriers against *Shigella* during storage.

Supplementary Materials: The following are available online at http://www.mdpi.com/2311-5637/5/2/34/s1, Table S1: Antagonistic activity of *L. rhamnosus* GG fortified sea buckthorn (SBT) and apple juice (APJ) against *Shigella dysteneriae* during 14 days storage, Table S2: Antagonistic activity of *L. rhamnosus* GG fortified sea buckthorn (SBT) and apple juice (APJ) against *Shigella flexneri* during 14 days storage.

Author Contributions: G.D. conceived and designed the experiments; S.S. performed the experiments and analyzed the data; Department of Science and Technology (DST) provided reagents/materials/analysis tools; S.S. and G.D. wrote the paper. D.M. provided his expert comments during the manuscript preparation.

Acknowledgments: The work was funded under the project No.: SEED/TSP/CODER/008/2012.

Conflicts of Interest: The authors declare no conflict of interest.

References

1. Platts-Mills, J.A.; Babji, S.; Bodhidatta, L.; Gratz, J.; Haque, R.; Havt, A.; McCormick, B.J.; McGrath, M.; Olortegui, M.P.; Samie, A.; et al. Pathogen-specific burdens of community diarrhoea in developing countries: A multisite birth cohort study (MAL-ED). *Lancet Glob. Health* **2015**, *3*, e564–e575. [CrossRef]
2. GBD. Disease and Injury Incidence and Prevalence Collaborators. Global, regional, and national incidence, prevalence, and years lived with disability for 310 acute and chronic diseases and injuries, 1990–2015: A systematic analysis for the Global Burden of Disease Study 2015. *Lancet* **2016**, *388*, 1545–1602.
3. Kotloff, K.L. The burden and etiology of diarrheal illness in developing countries. *Pediatr. Clin. N. Am.* **2017**, *64*, 799–814. [CrossRef] [PubMed]
4. Niyogi, S.K. Shigellosis. *J. Microbiol.* **2005**, *43*, 133–143. [PubMed]
5. Sur, D.; Ramamurthy, T.; Deen, J.; Bhattacharya, S.K. Shigellosis: Challenges & management issues. *Indian J. Med. Res.* **2004**, *20*, 454–462.
6. Greenhill, C. Diarrhoea: Tackling the problem of moderate-to-severe diarrhoea in developing countries. *Nat. Rev. Gastroenterol. Hepatol.* **2013**, *10*, 384–385. [CrossRef] [PubMed]
7. Rabaa, M.A.; Thanh, D.P.; De Lappe, N.; Cormican, M.; Valcanis, M.; Howden, B.P.; Wangchuk, S.; Bodhidatta, L.; Mason, C.J.; Nguyen, T.N.; et al. South Asia as a reservoir for the global spread of ciprofloxacin-resistant *Shigella sonnei*: A cross-sectional study. *PLoS Med.* **2016**, *13*, e1002055. [CrossRef]
8. Livio, S.; Strockbine, N.A.; Panchalingam, S.; Tennant, S.M.; Barry, E.M.; Marohn, M.E.; Antonio, M.; Hossain, A.; Mandomando, I.; Ochieng, J.B.; et al. Shigella isolates from the global enteric multicenter study inform vaccine development. *Clin. Infect. Dis.* **2014**, *59*, 933–941. [CrossRef] [PubMed]
9. Kim, H.J.; Youn, S.K.; Lee, S.; Choi, Y.H. Epidemiological Characteristics of Imported Shigellosis in Korea, 2010–2011. *Osong Public Health Res. Perspect.* **2013**, *4*, 159–165. [CrossRef] [PubMed]
10. Kosek, M.; Yori, P.P.; Olortegui, M.P. Shigellosis update: Advancing antibiotic resistance, investment empowered vaccine development, and green bananas. *Curr. Opin. Infect. Dis.* **2017**, *23*, 475–480. [CrossRef] [PubMed]

11. Jernberg, C.; Löfmark, S.; Edlund, C.; Jansson, J.K. Long-term impacts of antibiotic exposure on the human intestinal microbiota. *Microbiology* **2010**, *156*, 3216–3223. [CrossRef] [PubMed]
12. Narayan, S.S.; Jalgaonkar, S.; Shahani, S.; Kulkarni, V.N. Probiotics: Current trends in the treatment of diarrhoea. *Hong Kong Med. J.* **2010**, *16*, 213–218. [PubMed]
13. Hemarajata, P.; Versalovic, J. Effects of probiotics on gut microbiota: Mechanisms of intestinal immunomodulation and neuromodulation. *Therap. Adv. Gastroenterol.* **2013**, *6*, 39–51. [CrossRef] [PubMed]
14. Tejero-Sariñena, S.; Barlow, J.; Costabile, A.; Gibson, G.R.; Rowland, I. In vitro evaluation of the antimicrobial activity of a range of probiotics against pathogens: Evidence for the effects of organic acids. *Anaerobe* **2012**, *18*, 530–538. [CrossRef] [PubMed]
15. Davoodabadi, A.; Dallal, M.M.; Foroushani, A.R.; Douraghi, M.; Harati, F.A. Antibacterial activity of *Lactobacillus* spp. isolated from the feces of healthy infants against enteropathogenic bacteria. *Anaerobe* **2015**, *34*, 53–58. [CrossRef] [PubMed]
16. Zhang, Y.; Zhang, L.; Du, M.; Yi, H.; Guo, C.; Tuo, Y.; Han, X.; Li, J.; Zhang, L.; Yang, L. Antimicrobial activity against *Shigella sonnei* and probiotic properties of wild lactobacilli from fermented food. *Microbiol. Res.* **2011**, *167*, 27–31. [CrossRef] [PubMed]
17. Kakisu, E.; Bolla, P.; Abraham, A.G.; De Urraza, P.; de Antoni, G.L. *Lactobacillus plantarum* isolated from kefir: Protection of cultured Hep-2 cells against Shigella invasion. *Int. Dairy J.* **2013**, *33*, 22–26. [CrossRef]
18. Carlson, J.; Slavin, J. Health benefits of fibre, prebiotics and probiotics: A review of intestinal health and related health claims. *Qual. Assur. Saf. Crop* **2016**, *8*, 539–554. [CrossRef]
19. Tripathi, M.K.; Giri, S.K. Probiotic functional foods: Survival of probiotics during processing and storage. *J. Funct. Foods* **2014**, *9*, 225–241. [CrossRef]
20. Galgano, F.; Condelli, N.; Caruso, M.C.; Colangelo, M.A.; Favati, F. Probiotics and prebiotics in fruits and vegetables: Technological and sensory aspects. In *Beneficial Microbes in Fermented and Functional Foods*; CRC Press-Taylor & Francis Group: Abingdon, UK, 2014; pp. 189–206.
21. Güler-Akın, M.B.; Ferliarslan, I.; Akın, M.S. Apricot probiotic drinking yoghurt supplied with inulin and oat fiber. *Adv. Microbiol.* **2016**, *6*, 999–1009. [CrossRef]
22. Homayoni Rad, A.; Vaghef Mehrabany, E.; Alipoor, B.; Vaghef Mehrabany, L. The comparison of food and supplement as probiotic delivery vehicles. *Crit. Rev. Food Sci. Nutr.* **2016**, *56*, 896–909. [CrossRef] [PubMed]
23. Alwis, A.D.P.S.; Perera, O.D.A.N.; Weerahewa, H.L.D. Development of a Novel Carrot-based Synbiotic Beverage using *Lactobacillus casei* 431®. *J. Agric. Sci.* **2016**, *11*, 178–185. [CrossRef]
24. Di Cagno, R.; Coda, R.; De Angelis, M.; Gobbetti, M. Exploitation of vegetables and fruits through lactic acid fermentation. *Food Microbiol.* **2013**, *33*, 1–10. [CrossRef] [PubMed]
25. Alves, N.N.; Messaoud, G.B.; Desobry, S.; Costa, J.M.C.; Rodrigues, S. Effect of drying technique and feed flow rate on bacterial survival and physicochemical properties of a non-dairy fermented probiotic juice powder. *J. Food Eng.* **2016**, *189*, 45–54. [CrossRef]
26. Dharmasena, M.; Barron, F.; Fraser, A.; Jiang, X. Refrigerated Shelf Life of a Coconut Water-Oatmeal Mix and the Viability of Lactobacillus Plantarum Lp 115-400B. *Foods* **2015**, *4*, 328–337. [CrossRef] [PubMed]
27. Valero-Cases, E.; Nuncio-Jáuregui, N.; Frutos, M.J. Influence of fermentation with different lactic acid bacteria and in vitro digestion on the biotransformation of phenolic compounds in fermented pomegranate juices. *J. Agric. Food Chem.* **2017**, *65*, 6488–6496. [CrossRef] [PubMed]
28. Cardona, F.; Andrés-Lacueva, C.; Tulipani, S.; Tinahones, F.J.; Queipo-Ortuño, M.I. Benefits of polyphenols on gut microbiota and implications in human health. *J. Nutr. Biochem.* **2013**, *24*, 1415–1422. [CrossRef] [PubMed]
29. Gyawali, R.; Ibrahim, S.A. Impact of plant derivatives on the growth of foodborne pathogens and the functionality of probiotics. *Appl. Microbiol. Biotechnol.* **2012**, *95*, 29–45. [CrossRef] [PubMed]
30. Wishon, L.M.; Song, D.; Ibrahim, S. Effect of metals on growth and functionality of *Lactobacillus* and *Bifidobacteria*. *Milchwissenschaft* **2010**, *65*, 369–372.
31. Sireswar, S.; Dey, G.; Sreesoundarya, T.K.; Sarkar, D. Design of probiotic-fortified food matrices influence their antipathogenic potential. *Food Biosci.* **2017**, *20*, 28–35. [CrossRef]
32. Sireswar, S.; Dey, G.; Dey, K.; Kundu, A. Evaluation of Probiotic *L. rhamnosus* GG as a Protective Culture in Sea Buckthorn-Based Beverage. *Beverages* **2017**, *3*, 48. [CrossRef]
33. Singleton, V.L.; Orthofer, R.; Lamuela-Raventós, R.M. Analysis of total phenols and other oxidation substrates and antioxidants by means of Folin-Ciocalteu reagent. *Methods Enzymol.* **1999**, *299*, 152–178. [CrossRef]

34. Sánchez-Maldonado, A.F.; Schieber, A.; Gänzle, M.G. Structure–function relationships of the antibacterial activity of phenolic acids and their metabolism by lactic acid bacteria. *J. Appl. Microbiol.* **2011**, *11*, 1176–1184. [CrossRef] [PubMed]
35. Gunenc, A.; Khoury, C.; Legault, C.; Mirrashed, H.; Rijke, J.; Hosseinian, F. Seabuckthorn as a novel prebiotic source improves probiotic viability in yogurt. *LWT-Food Sci. Technol.* **2016**, *66*, 490–495. [CrossRef]
36. Terpou, A.; Gialleli, A.I.; Bosnea, L.; Kanellaki, M.; Koutinas, A.A.; Castro, G.R. Novel cheese production by incorporation of sea buckthorn berries (*Hippophae rhamnoides* L.) supported probiotic cells. *LWT-Food Sci. Technol.* **2017**, *79*, 616–624. [CrossRef]
37. Arora, R.; Mundra, S.; Yadav, A.; Srivastava, R.B.; Stobdan, T. Antimicrobial activity of seed, pomace and leaf extracts of sea buckthorn (*Hippophae rhamnoides* L.) against foodborne and food spoilage pathogens. *Afr. J. Biotechnol.* **2012**, *11*, 10424–10430. [CrossRef]
38. Van Opstal, I.; Bagamboula, C.F.; Theys, T.; Vanmuysen, S.C.M.; Michiels, C.W. Inactivation of Escherichia coli and *Shigella* in acidic fruit and vegetable juices by peroxidase systems. *J. Appl Microbiol.* **2006**, *101*, 242–250. [CrossRef] [PubMed]
39. Vinderola, G.; Binetti, A.; Burns, P.; Reinheimer, J. Cell viability and functionality of probiotic bacteria in dairy products. *Front. Microbiol.* **2011**, *2*, 1–6. [CrossRef] [PubMed]
40. Madureira, A.R.; Amorim, M.; Gomes, A.M.; Pintado, M.E.; Malcata, F.X. Protective effect of whey cheese matrix on probiotic strains exposed to simulated gastrointestinal conditions. *Food Res. Int.* **2011**, *44*, 465–470. [CrossRef]
41. In, Y.W.; Kim, J.J.; Kim, H.J.; Oh, S.W. Antimicrobial activities of acetic acid, citric acid and lactic acid against Shigella species. *J. Food Saf.* **2013**, *33*, 79–85. [CrossRef]
42. Bagamboula, C.F.; Uyttendaele, M.; Debevere, J. Acid tolerance of *Shigella sonnei* and *Shigella flexneri*. *J. Appl. Microbiol.* **2002**, *93*, 479–486. [CrossRef] [PubMed]
43. Yang, G.; Wang, L.; Wang, Y.; Li, P.; Zhu, J.; Qiu, S.; Hao, R.; Wu, Z.; Li, W.; Song, H. hfq regulates acid tolerance and virulence by responding to acid stress in *Shigella flexneri*. *Res. Microbiol.* **2015**, *166*, 166–476. [CrossRef] [PubMed]
44. Lacombe, A.; Wu, V.C.; White, J.; Tadepalli, S.; Andre, E.E. The antimicrobial properties of the lowbush blueberry (*Vaccinium angustifolium*) fractional components against foodborne pathogens and the conservation of probiotic Lactobacillus rhamnosus. *Food Microbiol.* **2012**, *30*, 124–131. [CrossRef] [PubMed]
45. Rodrıguez, E.; Calzada, J.; Arqués, J.L.; Rodrıguez, J.M.; Nunez, M.; Medina, M. Antimicrobial activity of pediocin-producing *Lactococcus lactis* on *Listeria monocytogenes*, *Staphylococcus aureus* and *Escherichia coli* O157: H7 in cheese. *Int. Dairy J.* **2005**, *15*, 51–57. [CrossRef]
46. McAuliffe, O.; Hill, C.; Ross, R.P. Inhibition of *Listeria monocytogenes* in cottage cheese manufactured with a lacticin 3147-producing starter culture. *J. Appl. Microbiol.* **1999**, *86*, 251–256. [CrossRef] [PubMed]
47. Arqués, J.L.; Rodríguez, E.; Gaya, P.; Medina, M.; Guamis, B.; Nunez, M. Inactivation of *Staphylococcus aureus* in raw milk cheese by combinations of high-pressure treatments and bacteriocin-producing lactic acid bacteria. *J. Appl. Microbiol.* **2005**, *98*, 254–260. [CrossRef] [PubMed]

© 2018 by the authors. Licensee MDPI, Basel, Switzerland. This article is an open access article distributed under the terms and conditions of the Creative Commons Attribution (CC BY) license (http://creativecommons.org/licenses/by/4.0/).

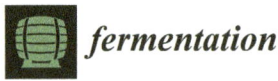

Article

The Effect of Salt and Temperature on the Growth of Fresco Culture

Alžbeta Medveďová *, Petra Šipošová, Tatiana Mančušková and Ľubomír Valík

Department of Nutrition and Food Quality Assessment, Faculty of Chemical and Food Technology, Slovak, University of Technology, Radlinského 9, 81237 Bratislava, Slovakia; petra.siposova@stuba.sk (P.Š.); tatiana.mancuskova@stuba.sk (T.M.); lubomir.valik@stuba.sk (Ľ.V.)
* Correspondence: alzbeta.medvedova@stuba.sk; Tel.: + 421-2-59325-524

Received: 26 October 2018; Accepted: 17 December 2018; Published: 20 December 2018

Abstract: The effect of environmental factors, including temperature and water activity, has a considerable impact on the growth dynamics of each microbial species, and it is complicated in the case of mixed cultures. Therefore, the aim of this study was to describe and analyze the growth dynamics of Fresco culture (consisting of 3 different bacterial species) using predictive microbiology tools. The growth parameters from primary fitting were modelled against temperature using two different secondary models. The intensity of Fresco culture growth in milk was significantly affected by incubation temperature described by Gibson's model, from which the optimal temperature for growth of 38.6 °C in milk was calculated. This cardinal temperature was verified with the T_{opt} = 38.3 °C calculated by the CTMI model (cardinal temperature model with inflection), providing other cardinal temperatures, i.e., minimal T_{min} = 4.0 °C and maximal T_{max} = 49.6 °C for Fresco culture growth. The specific growth rate of the culture under optimal temperature was 1.56 h^{-1}. The addition of 1% w/v salt stimulated the culture growth dynamics under temperatures down to 33 °C but not the rate of milk acidification. The prediction data were validated and can be used in dairy practice during manufacture of fermented dairy products.

Keywords: fresco culture; growth parameters; predictive microbiology

1. Introduction

Predictive microbiology is a very useful approach to characterize the growth of microorganisms in relation to selected environmental factors. The fundamentals for predictive microbiology were derived in 1949 from the Monod's definition according to which "the growth of bacterial cultures, despite the immense complexity of the phenomena to which it testifies, generally obeys relatively simple laws". Thus, the responses of a microbial population to environmental factors are reproducible [1]. Predictive microbiology would not only enable us to focus on foodborne and spoilage microorganisms but it should also predict the behavior of starter cultures during fermentation, at least of dairy products [2,3].

In milk fermentations, lactic acid bacteria (LAB) are the dominant microbiota. Their metabolic activity leads to desired degradation of saccharides, lipids, proteins and other milk components forming a wide range of metabolites, which have a positive effect on the technological and sensory properties of the final product [4–6]. The products obtained by their use are characterized by increased hygienic safety, prolonged storage stability and more attractive sensory properties [7]. Another positive feature of some LAB is their ability to improve or maintain the good health of consumers [8]. It is also important that LAB have a great ability to enter associative relationships in mixed cultures, since the symbiotic interrelationships among microbiota are of fundamental importance in food fermentation. The growth and metabolism of some LAB strains may be stimulated by another LAB member, particularly under environmental conditions, where one or both bacteria are not able to grow without the other [9,10]. Therefore, the choice of an appropriate active starter culture for controlled fermentation processes is of utmost importance [11]. Moreover, the growth and metabolism of microorganisms, alone or in mixed populations, are affected by many intrinsic (e.g., salt addition) and extrinsic (e.g., temperature) factors. Sensitivity of bacterial cultures to actual salt addition is strongly dependent on bacterial species and strain, and therefore the salt concentration can have stimulating or inhibiting effects on bacterial metabolic activity. One of the starter cultures used in cheese technology, e.g., in Mozzarella type or Cottage cheese production [4,12] is also Fresco DVS 1010 culture consisting of 3 different species—*Lactococcus lactis* ssp. *lactis*, able to grow at up to 4% of NaCl, *Lc. lactis* ssp. *cremoris*, able to grow at up to 2% of NaCl and *Streptococcus salivarius* ssp. *thermophilus*, able to grow at 2.5% NaCl [13].

Since the temperature and salt concentration are among the most important factors for bioprocess control, a description of the effect of temperature and water activity on the microbial growth parameters is required. That is why this work deals with the quantification of the effect that temperature and salt addition have on the growth of Fresco DVS 1010 culture. Mathematical modelling coupled with experimental analysis allows us to understand the growth dynamics of studied mixed culture under specific conditions. These data will help optimize the process of cheese manufacturing conditions when a mixed culture of LAB will be used as a starter culture.

2. Materials and Methods

2.1. Microorganisms

Fresco DVS 1010 culture (Fresco culture; Christian Hansen, Hørsholm, Denmark) consisting of *Lactococcus lactis* subsp. *lactis*, *Lc. lactis* subsp. *cremoris* and *Streptococcus salivarius* ssp. *thermophilus* was used. This commercial culture was kept frozen at −40 °C until use.

2.2. Inoculation and Cultivation Conditions

A few grains of the frozen Fresco culture were inoculated into 100 mL of sterile milk and incubated at 30 °C for 5 h until the stationary phase was reached. Appropriate dilutions of this culture were used to inoculate 300 mL of pre-tempered ultra-pasteurized milk (1.5 g/L fat content, Rajo, Bratislava, Slovakia) so that the initial concentration was as close as possible to 10^4 CFU/mL. The incubation was performed in three parallel stages under static conditions at appropriately chosen temperatures in the range from 5 to 47 °C.

2.3. The Effect of NaCl Addition on the Growth of Fresco Culture

The effect of NaCl addition (1, 2 and 3%, w/v) was studied in milk (1.5 g/L fat content, Rajo, Bratislava, Slovakia) at temperatures of 12, 15, 18, 21, 25, 30 and 37 °C in three parallel stages. The conditions of inoculation (initial counts of approximately 10^3 CFU/mL) were mentioned above. The value of water activity was controlled by an a_w-meter (Aw-Sprint TH500, Novasina, Lachen, Switzerland).

2.4. Total Counts of Fresco Culture in Growth Media

At chosen time intervals, the number of bacteria in the culture was determined according to EN ISO 4833-1 [14] on M17 agar (Biokar Diagnostics, Beauvais, France).

2.5. Fitting the Growth Curves and Calculating the Growth Parameters

The growth data of Fresco culture were analyzed, fitted and calculated, using DMFit Excel Add-in package version 3.5 (ComBase managed by United States Department of Agriculture-Agricultural Research Service, Washington, DC, USA and University of Tasmania Food Safety Centre Hobart, Australia) that incorporates the mechanistic modeling technique of Baranyi and Roberts [15]. The counts were plotted against time and fitted to a model for the estimation of the growth rate (Gr), the initial (N_0) and maximal (N_{max}) density. The growth parameters from the individual parallel experiments were analyzed in the secondary phase of modeling by statistical tools of the Microsoft Office version 2007 (Microsoft, Redmond, WA, USA) and the Statistica data analysis software system, version 8.0 (StatSoft, Inc., Tulsa, OK, USA).

2.6. Secondary Models

To empirically describe the influence of selected environmental factor on the data in the whole temperature range, the cardinal temperature model with inflection (CTMI) was introduced. This model uses three cardinal temperatures directly included as parameters of the model. Its advantage is the direct definition of cardinal temperature values for the growth of selected bacteria [16]. The effect of temperature on the specific growth rate ($\mu = \ln 10 \times Gr$) is described by the equations:

$$\mu = \mu_{opt} \frac{a}{b * c} \quad (1)$$

$$a = (T - T_{max})(T - T_{min})^2, \quad b = (T_{opt} - T_{min})$$
$$c = (T_{opt} - T_{min})(T - T_{min}) - (T_{opt} - T_{max})(T_{opt} + T_{min} - 2T)$$

where T is actual incubation temperature, T_{min} is the notional temperature below which the growth is not observed, T_{max} is the notional temperature above which the growth is not observed and T_{opt} is the temperature at which the maximal growth (Gr_{opt}) is observed [16].

The specific growth rate (μ) was also modeled as a function of the incubation temperature T by the model introduced by Gibson et al. [17]. Again, the maximal specific growth rate was modeled as a function of the incubation temperature. For that purpose and inspired by the water activity (a_w) transformation originally introduced by Gibson et al. [17], the following transformation of temperature (T_w) was applied.

$$T_w = \sqrt{(T_{max} - T)} \quad (2)$$

T_{max} was given by the CTMI model and was also confirmed by the estimation from data points in the high-temperature region as recommended by Ratkowsky et al. [18]. The natural logarithm of the specific growth rates was modeled by the following quadratic function as introduced by Gibson et al. [17]:

$$\ln \mu = C_0 + C_1 T_w + C_2 T_w^2 \quad (3)$$

The coefficients C_0, C_1 and C_2 were estimated by linear regression. Finally, the optimum value $T_{opt} = T_{max} - (C_1/C_2)^2$ for the maximal growth rate was calculated.

The same models were used for the prediction of Fresco culture growth dynamics at selected NaCl concentrations as a function of temperature.

2.7. Validation of the Models

To validate the mathematical equations describing Fresco culture responses to various environmental conditions, several mathematical and statistical indices were used. The ordinary least-squares criterion and regression coefficient (R^2) were used to describe the fit of the model to the data. The variance percentage (%V) as given by Daughtry et al. [19] gives the goodness of the fit of the model; the root mean square error (RMSE) as given by TeGiffel & Zwietering [20] as well as the sum of the squared residuals (RSS) as reported Zwietering et al. [21] and standard error of prediction (%SEP) as reported Zurera-Cosano et al. [22] were used as a measure of "goodness-of-fit". Finally, accuracy (Af), bias (Bf) and discrepancy (Df) factors as introduced by Baranyi et al. [23] were used for internal validation of the models.

3. Results

To describe the effect of the incubation temperature on Fresco culture growth, experiments were carried out in the ultra-pasteurised milk. The average initial counts of Fresco culture (N_0) in all experiments were 4.30 ± 0.39 log CFU/mL (%V = 9.0). All growth curves were characterized by a typical sigmoidal shape and were successfully fitted with the model of Baranyi & Roberts [15] with R^2 = 0.994 ± 0.006. The temperature of 5 °C was the minimal temperature at which the growth of the culture was noticed, though the growth was very slow, represented by time to double of 30.6 h where $t_d = ln2/\mu$ [23]. Further increase in temperature led to more and more intensive growth of bacterial populations. Comparing the growth rate at 7, 10, 12 and 15 °C, the intensity of multiplication increased about 70%, 38%, 27% and 50% in comparison to growth rate at 5 °C. This almost linear trend continued until 40 °C, when the fastest growth of Gr = 0.961 log CFU/mL·h^{-1} was reached. Further increase of the incubation temperature had a negative effect on the growth dynamics, since the growth rate decreased to Gr = 0.582 log CFU/mL·h^{-1} at 43 °C and Gr = 0.349 log CFU/mL·h^{-1} at 47 °C.

Although the growth dynamics were strongly influenced by the incubation temperature; the growth increment and the final densities of Fresco culture were constant even at low temperatures. At the lowest temperature, the stationary phase was reached after almost 27 days (674 h); on the other hand, at 40 °C the stationary phase was reached only after 8 h of incubation. It is important to note that the average counts in the stationary phase of N_{max} = 8.85 ± 0.44 log CFU/mL (%V = 4.9) were reached at all studied temperatures. On the other hand, during the growth of some lactic acid bacteria as a monoculture, e.g., *Lactobacillus rhamnosus* GG [24], *Lb. acidophilus* NCFM Howaru [25] or *Lb. plantarum* [26] strong influence of temperature on the final number of bacterial cells was observed. The cause might be Fresco being a mixed culture, since Champagne et al. [27] noticed about 20% increase in growth of cells and about 13% higher growth dynamics of *Lc. lactis* in the presence of *S. thermophilus* compared to growth of lactococci alone. On the other hand, growth increment and growth dynamics of *S. thermophilus* were not influenced by the presence of *Lc. lactis*. We supposed that bacterial partners did not compete for nutrients at the same time. Moreover, thanks to the metabolism and subsequent production of substrates needed for the growth of the second bacterial partner, its growth might be stimulated.

3.1. The Effect of Incubation Temperature on Fresco Culture Growth Rate

From the primary growth curves of Fresco culture in milk, the growth rate Gr (expressed as the logarithm of colony forming units per millilitre and per hour) or the specific growth rate μ (expressed as reciprocal hours) was derived from 3 replicate curves at each temperature, and values are summarized in Table 1. Individual data were subsequently used in the secondary phase of predictive modeling and graphical presentations. Each part of the growth curve was also influenced by environmental factors or conditions prior to growth analysis, so the secondary models represent an essential approach to describe the influence of selected factors on microbial growth.

To predict the effect of the incubation temperature on the growth dynamics of Fresco culture in milk, an empirical CTMI model was used. Since the parameter settings of the CTMI model are based on their biological interpretation and due to the lack of structural correlation between parameters, the simple and accurate estimation of cardinal temperature values is allowed [16]. The most optimal conditions for Fresco culture growth in milk are expected at 38.3 °C. Under the optimal temperature conditions, the 4th parameter of the CTMI model provides the maximal specific growth rate of 1.56 h^{-1}. This can be used by dairy technologists and microbiologists in dairy practice after its recalculation to time to doubling time and it is expected to be 26.7 min in milk.

Table 1. Effect of temperature on the growth and metabolic activity of Fresco culture in milk.

T	Gr	λ	N_{max}	r_{pH}	lag_{pH}
5	0.010 ± 0.001	146.8 ± 8.96	8.94 ± 0.06	−0.033	547.0
7	0.032 ± 0.001	43.0 ± 4.44	8.17 ± 0.02	−0.004	130.0
12	0.071 ± 0.007	3.4 ± 0.17	8.87 ± 0.09	−0.053	54.3
15	0.140 ± 0.011	6.7 ± 1.80	9.26 ± 0.05	−0.048	24.1
18	0.196 ± 0.001	4.2 ± 0.10	8.97 ± 0.03	−0.087	19.9
21	0.257 ± 0.000	-	9.33 ± 0.02	−0.308	17.3
25	0.390 ± 0.008	1.2 ± 0.02	9.27 ± 0.14	−0.324	7.9
31	0.567 ± 0.008	2.2 ± 0.04	9.35 ± 0.05	−0.612	9.7
37	0.722 ± 0.027	0.5 ± 0.05	8.59 ± 0.05	−0.451	4.5
40	0.961 ± 0.217	1.87 ± 0.54	8.68 ± 0.07	−0.234	12.3
43	0.582 ± 0.019	0.8 ± 0.08	8.40 ± 0.21	−0.381	7.5
47	0.349 ± 0.018	-	7.90 ± 0.21	−0.070	-

T—Incubation temperature (°C), Gr—growth rate (log CFU/mL·h^{-1}), λ—lag phase duration (h), N_{max}—counts of Fresco culture in the stationary phase (log CFU/mL), r_{pH}—rate of pH value decrease (h^{-1}), lag_{pH}—lag of pH value (h).

By using the CTMI model (Figure 1), the other cardinal temperatures were estimated: minimal temperature (below which no growth occurs) is 4.0 °C, maximal temperature allowing growth is 49.6 °C. These findings also confirmed that our estimations of the maximal temperature of 49 °C based on the recommendation of Ratkowsky et al. [18] needed for Gibson's model were sufficiently precise. With respect to different modeling techniques, the narrow range of each cardinal temperature for Fresco culture is expected with defined errors in expectation, considering the discrepancies calculated in the validation process that is an inevitable part of the mathematical prediction of microbial growth under specific environmental conditions.

The estimation of optimal temperature for growth of Fresco culture was also confirmed by Gibson's model with the temperature transformation (Equation (3)). The specific growth rate of Fresco culture was plotted against calculated T_w values (Equation (2)) and was fitted with a regression model (Equation (4)) with good fitting in the range beyond T_{opt} (R^2 = 0.984).

$$ln\mu = -2.4192 + 1.8916T_w + 0.2929T_w^2 \qquad (4)$$

Based on this equation, the optimal temperature of T_{opt} = 38.6 °C for Fresco culture growth in milk was calculated, which is in perfect agreement with the optimal temperature calculated by the CTMI model. From the food practice point of view, predictive microbiology can provide some easily interpretable data, such as how fast microorganisms grow in a given product or when the stationary phase will be reached. The prediction of time necessary to increase culture density at the selected temperature of the process is a main concern for food technologists. That is why the predictions of the time (t_x) needed for increase of Fresco culture in milk regarding x logarithmic counts (x = 1, 2, ...) at a selected temperature can be a useful application of Gibson's model. In this approach it was assumed that time t_x is inversely related to the growth kinetic ($ln\ \mu$) described by the model according to the equation $ln\ t_x = x/\mu$, where $\mu = exp^{(-2.4192 + 1.8916T_w + 0.2929T_w^2)}$.

It is also important to mention the desirable function of lactic acid bacteria, i.e., their inhibitive potential against some bacteria. During raw milk fermentation, coagulase-positive staphylococci, pathogenic or saprophytic *Escherichia coli* are the most frequent undesirable species with highly adverse health effect on consumers. In our previous works [28–30], we proved that Fresco culture has strong inhibitive potential against *Staphylococcus aureus* or *Escherichia coli* growth in milk co-culture and did not influence the growth of *Geotrichum candidum* that might play an important role during fresh cheese ripening [30].

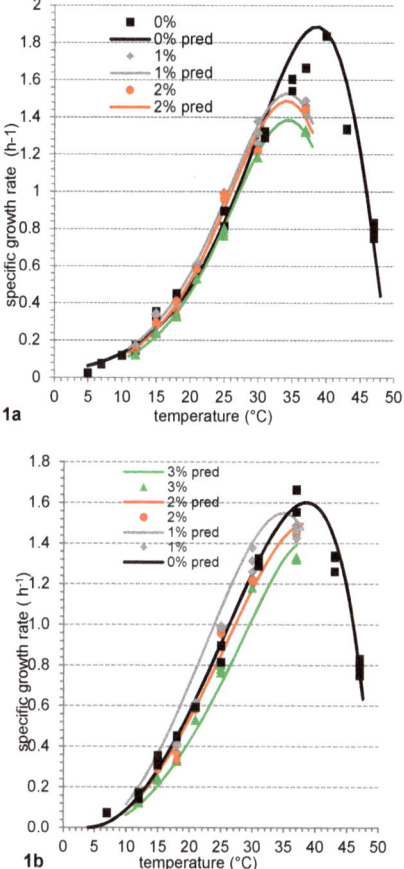

Figure 1. Plots of the specific growth rates (μ) versus temperature (T) for Fresco culture in milk according to (**a**) Gibson's model and (**b**) CTMI model (solid line). Symbols indicate the μ calculated from the growth curves at each incubation temperature. The continuous lines indicate the fitted μ versus T function according to each model for 0% (■), 1% (♦), 2% (●) and 3% (▲) of salt.

3.2. The Effect of NaCl on the Growth Dynamics of Fresco Culture

Besides the growth of Fresco culture in milk without additional salt (a_w = 0.995 ± 0.002; %V = 1.9), the effect of 1% (1 g/100 mL) salt addition (a_w = 0.992 ± 0.001; %V = 0.11), 2% (2 g/100 mL) NaCl addition (a_w = 0.987 ± 0.003; %V = 0.28) and 3% (3 g/100 mL) NaCl addition (a_w = 0.979 ± 0.002; %V = 0.21) was studied at temperatures 12, 15, 18, 21, 25, 30 and 37 °C. All growth curves were again characterized by a typical sigmoid shape and were successfully fitted with the model of Baranyi & Roberts [15] at R^2 = 0.997 ± 0.003.

The growth dynamics of Fresco culture were stimulated by the 1% salt addition as was seen by a higher growth rate as well as by a shorter lag phase duration. However, a further increase in the salt concentration in the media led to the deceleration of Fresco culture growth. It is apparent from both Gibson's model (Figure 1a) as well as the CTMI model (Figure 1b). However, this stimulation of growth dynamics by 1% salt addition was observed only at temperatures below 33 °C. At 37 °C, Fresco culture grew about 20% slower in media with 1% salt addition compared to the control. However, 2 or 3% addition of NaCl led generally to a lowering of Fresco culture growth dynamics. Liu et al. [31] observed slowing of *Lc. lactis* ssp. *cremoris* 2260 growth in M17 broth at 22 °C by about 33% in media with a_w = 0.98 compared to media without the salt addition. In the case of our studies, Fresco culture grew at 21 °C about 10% slower in media with a_w = 0.977 compared to media without salt addition. This might be the result of the presence of compatible solutes (carnitine, betaine, proline, etc.) in milk [32] that protect Fresco culture to withstand unfavorable environmental conditions. Similarly, Uguen et al. [33] observed slowing of Lc. lactis ssp. lactis ADRIA 85LO30 growth, approximately 3-fold, in the presence of 23.4 g/L of NaCl while the addition of osmoprotective compounds (betaine, dimethylsulfonioacetate, dimethylsulfoniopropionate, L-carnitine) into the same media with 23.4 g/L NaCl led to slowing of the growth dynamics but only by about 24%.

Use of lactic acid bacteria starter culture is limited not only by their growth activity but also by their fast acidification activity that is also influenced by many intrinsic and extrinsic factors. During growth of Fresco culture in milk, the slowest pH value decline was observed naturally at the lowest temperatures and at the highest salt addition. At higher incubation temperatures, the rate of pH value decrease (r_{pH}) was more intensive as can be seen from Tables 1 and 2. However, as the salt concentration increased, the rate of pH change decreased and the lag phase of pH change was longer, even when the differences at 1% of salt concentration were not so dramatic. Larsen & Añón [34] noticed that even though the growth of S. thermophilus ATCC 19258 was not influenced by the presence of glycerol, the acidification ability was slowed down by about 10% compared to the acidification rate in media without glycerol. Moreover, Liu et al. [31] observed that by decreasing water activity value from 0.99 to 0.88, the acidification rate of Lc. lactis ssp. cremoris 2254 was lowered by 13.5 to 42.4%, depending on pH.

Table 2. The effect of temperature and water activity on the growth and metabolic activity of Fresco culture in milk.

T	a_w	Gr	λ	N_{max}	r_{pH}	lag_{pH}
	0.991	0.074 ± 0.000	3.8 ± 0.1	9.36 ± 0.01	−0.175	101.2
12	0.987	0.064 ± 0.000	7.7 ± 0.2	9.11 ± 0.04	−0.101	112.2
	0.981	0.054 ± 0.001	14.0 ± 1.4	9.13 ± 0.13	−0.040	116.3
	0.993	0.147 ± 0.002	3.5 ± 0.3	9.27 ± 0.03	−0.126	42.0
15	0.988	0.127 ± 0.003	4.1 ± 0.2	9.21 ± 0.08	−0.113	51.9
	0.981	0.105 ± 0.002	6.6 ± 0.0	9.15 ± 0.04	−0.075	63.4
	0.993	0.175 ± 0.002	0.2 ± 0.5	9.12 ± 0.06	−0.086	23.5
18	0.989	0.159 ± 0.017	2.0 ± 0.6	9.01 ± 0.06	−0.098	32.3
	0.981	0.145 ± 0.002	4.6 ± 0.6	8.61 ± 0.08	−0.056	38.7
	0.992	0.265 ± 0.001	0.7 ± 0.1	9.33 ± 0.02	−0.209	21.2
21	0.989	0.253 ± 0.001	1.0 ± 0.0	9.60 ± 0.01	−0.155	21.2
	0.977	0.231 ± 0.000	2.1 ± 0.0	9.09 ± 0.06	−0.358	32.4
	0.992	0.430 ± 0.002	1.2 ± 0.0	9.28 ± 0.00	−0.176	12.3
25	0.988	0.420 ± 0.008	1.8 ± 0.2	9.32 ± 0.00	−0.172	12.7
	0.977	0.342 ± 0.009	1.9 ± 0.1	8.91 ± 0.06	−0.132	18.4
	0.990	0.570 ± 0.019	0.4 ± 0.2	9.14 ± 0.11	−0.181	9.8
30	0.981	0.527 ± 0.011	0.1 ± 0.3	9.08 ± 0.26	−0.168	9.0
	0.977	0.514 ± 0.010	0.7 ± 0.3	9.17 ± 0.16	−0.182	11.2
	0.992	0.634 ± 0.014	0.3 ± 0.0	8.98 ± 0.02	−0.297	7.0
37	0.986	0.629 ± 0.003	0.6 ± 0.0	9.38 ± 0.02	−0.231	8.6
	0.980	0.576 ± 0.003	1.2 ± 0.0	8.72 ± 0.04	−0.178	12.1

T—Incubation temperature (°C), Gr—growth rate (log CFU/mL·h^{-1}), λ—lag phase duration (h), N_{max}—counts of Fresco culture in stationary phase (log CFU/mL), r_{pH} —rate of pH decrease (h^{-1}), lag_{pH}—lag of pH value (h).

3.3. Validation

As there was a lack of comparable growth data for Fresco culture in the literature, only an internal validation was performed. Obtained validation indices are summarized in Table 3. The accuracy indices for the model predictions compared to the original data of Fresco culture were from 1.055 to 1.146 for Gibson's model and from 1.070 to 1.193 for the CTMI model. As proposed by Ross et al. [35], the relative error in growth estimates under controlled laboratory conditions was expected to be around 10% per independent variable. Therefore, if the temperature was the only factor, the best expected accuracy factor was approximately 1.1. For other lactic acid bacteria, we found similar accuracy factors, e.g., Af of 1.09 1.16 for the growth of *Leuconostoc mesenteroides* in a broth culture [22], for the growth of *Lactobacillus rhamnosus* GG in milk, Af of 1.102–1.201 [36], for the growth of *Lactobacillus acidophilus* NCFM in milk and in MRS broth, accuracy factor of 1.188–1.256 [25].

Table 3. The equations of Gibson's model, the coefficients of the CTMI model and the indices of the internal validation for Fresco culture growth.

	\multicolumn{8}{c}{Equation/Coefficients of the Equation}							
	Af	Bf	$\%Df$	R^2	$\%V$	RSS	RMSE	$\%SEP$
CTMI model								
0 %	1.070	0.995	7.0	0.987	98.3	0.069	0.051	6.1
1 %	1.193	1.156	19.3	0.949	93.3	0.231	0.093	12.3
2 %	1.090	0.987	9.0	0.985	98.0	0.067	0.049	6.9
3 %	1.134	0.904	13.4	0.949	93.1	0.185	0.083	13.3
	\multicolumn{8}{l}{Gibson's model $\ln \mu = -0.2929\, T_w^2 + 1.8916\, T_w - 2.4192$}							
0 %	1.146	1.010	14.6	0.984	98.3	0.129	0.058	16.1
	\multicolumn{8}{l}{Gibson's model $\ln \mu = -0.4165\, T_w^2 + 3.1904\, T_w - 5.6855$}							
1 %	1.082	0.999	8.2	0.988	98.6	0.032	0.039	5.2
	\multicolumn{8}{l}{Gibson's model $\ln \mu = -0.4447\, T_w^2 + 3.4149\, T_w - 6.1585$}							
2 %	1.090	0.999	9.0	0.987	98.5	0.060	0.055	8.0
	\multicolumn{8}{l}{Gibson's model $\ln \mu = -0.4522\, T_w^2 + 3.445\, T_w - 6.2354$}							
3 %	1.055	0.999	5.5	0.995	99.5	0.008	0.020	3.2

Except for the CTMI model at 1% and 3% of NaCl, all other applied models can be acceptable with high accuracy since, as proposed by Zurera-Cosano et al. [22], the model can be considered as good if the bias factor is in the range of 0.95–1.01. The bias factor higher than 1.0 (Gibson's model at 0% NaCl and CTMI at 1% NaCl) revealed overestimation of the growth rate that would lead to the slower real growth of Fresco culture in milk than is predicted by the models but with the defined errors expressed by the discrepancy factors. Taking the %Df and %SEP values into account, the predictions of growth rate of the culture can still be considered acceptable, since they range from 5.5 to 19.3 % in the case of %Df and from 3.2 to 16.1% in the case of %SEP. However, the well-thought interpretation of the obtained data is as important as their achievement.

4. Conclusions

In this work we studied the effect of temperature and salt concentration on the growth of mixed Fresco culture with the use of predictive models. Based on the models, the cardinal temperatures for Fresco culture growth were calculated and may be taken into account during dairy product manufacture and storage to ensure product stability and shelf-life. The addition of salt up to 1% stimulated the growth of Fresco culture, but not the rate of acidification of milk media. The inhibition of Fresco culture acidification was not significant and therefore the addition of salt can be used to inhibit pathogenic bacteria sensitive to lower water activity values. Moreover, all used models are suitable for the estimation of Fresco culture growth dynamics in dairy products and can be applied to increase storage stability and sensory attractiveness of products.

Author Contributions: P.Š., T.M. and A.M. were carried out the experimental work and analyzed the data, Ľ.V. set up the experimental design, A.M. and Ľ.V. wrote the paper.

Funding: This research was funded by grants VEGA No. 1/0532/18 and APVV-15-0006.

Acknowledgments: We would like to thank MSc. Michal Kaliňák for corrections.

Conflicts of Interest: The authors declare no conflict of interest.

References

1. Ross, T.; McMeekin, T.A. Predictive microbiology. *Int. J. Food Microbiol.* **1994**, *23*, 241–264. [CrossRef]
2. Aghababaie, M.; Khanahmadi, M.; Beheshti, M. Developing a detailed kinetic model for the production of yogurt starter bacteria in single strain cultures. *Food Bioprod. Process.* **2014**, *94*, 657–667. [CrossRef]
3. Alvarez, M.M.; Aguirre-Ezkauriatza, E.J.; Ramírez-Medrano, A.; Rodríguez-Sánchez, Á. Kinetic analysis and mathematical modeling of growth and lactic acid production of *Lactobacillus casei* var. *rhamnosus* in milk whey. *J. Dairy Sci.* **2010**, *93*, 5552–5560. [CrossRef] [PubMed]
4. Lahtinen, S.; Salminen, S.; Von Wright, A.; Ouwehand, A.C. *Lactic Acid Bacteria: Microbiological and Functional Aspects*, 4th ed.; CRC Press: Boca Raton, FL, USA, 2011; 779p, ISBN 978-1139836781.
5. Ljungh, A.; Wadström, T. *Lactobacillus Molecular Biology: From Genomics to Probiotics*, 1st ed.; Horizon Scientific Press: Norfolk, FL, USA, 2009; 205p, ISBN 978-1904455417.
6. Marth, E.C.; Steel, J.L. *Applied Dairy Microbiology*, 2nd ed.; Marcel Dekker, Inc.: New York, NY, USA, 2001; 736p, ISBN 978-0824705367.
7. Kavitake, D.; Kandasamy, S.; Devi, P.B.; Shetty, P.H. Recent developments on encapsulation of lactic acid bacteria as potential starter culture in fermented foods. *Food Biosci.* **2018**, *21*, 34–44. [CrossRef]
8. Mancuskova, T.; Medved'ova, A.; Ozbolt, M. The medical functions of probiotics and their role in clinical nutrition. *Curr. Nutr. Food Sci.* **2017**, *13*, 1–8. [CrossRef]
9. Sasaki, Y.; Horiuchi, H.; Kawashima, H.; Mukai, T.; Yamamoto, Y. NADH oxidase of *S. thermophilus* 1131 is required for the effective yogurt fermentation with *L. delbrueckii* subsp. *bulgaricus* 2038. *Biosci. Microbiota Food Health* **2014**, *33*, 31–40. [CrossRef]
10. Wang, T.; Xu, Z.; Lu, S.; Xin, M.; Kong, J. Effects of glutathione on acid stress resistance and symbiosis between *S. thermophilus* and *L. delbrueckii* subsp. *bulgaricus*. *Int. Dairy J.* **2016**, *61*, 22–28. [CrossRef]
11. Neysens, P.; Messens, W.; De Wuyst, L. Effect of NaCl on growth and bacteriocin production by *L. amylovorus* DCE 471. *Int. J. Food Microbiol.* **2003**, *88*, 29–39. [CrossRef]
12. Fresco DVS 1010 Culture. Available online: www.chr-hansen.com/en (accessed on 25 May 2018).
13. Ramchandran, L.; Sanciolo, P.; Vasiljevic, T.; Broome, M.; Powell, I.; Diuke, M. Improving cell yield and lactic acid production of *L. lactis* ssp. *cremoris* by a novel submerged membrane fermentation process. *J. Membr. Sci.* **2012**, *403*, 179–187. [CrossRef]
14. EN ISO 4833-1:2013. In *Microbiology of the Food Chain—Horizontal Method for the Enumeration of Microorganisms—Part 1: Colony Count at 30 °C by the Pour Plate Technique*; International Organization for Standardization: Geneva, Switzerland, 2013; 13p.
15. Baranyi, J.; Roberts, T.A. A dynamic approach to predicting bacterial growth in food. *Int. J. Food Microbiol.* **1994**, *23*, 277–294. [CrossRef]
16. Rosso, L.; Lobry, J.; Flanders, J. Unexpected correlation between temperatures of microbial growth highlighted by new model. *J. Theor. Biol.* **1993**, *162*, 447–463. [CrossRef]
17. Gibson, A.; Baranyi, J.; Pitt, J.I.; Eyles, M.J.; Roberts, T.A. Predicting fungal growth—The effect of water activity on *A. flavus* and related species. *Int. J. Food Microbiol.* **1994**, *23*, 419–431. [CrossRef]
18. Ratkowsky, D.A.; Lowry, R.K.; McMeekin, T.A.; Stokes, A.N.; Chandler, R.E. Model for bacterial culture growth rate throughout the entire biokinetic temperature range. *J. Bacteriol.* **1983**, *154*, 1222–1226.
19. Daughtry, B.J.; Davey, K.R.; King, K.D. Temperature dependence of growth kinetics of food bacteria. *Food Microbiol.* **1997**, *14*, 21–30. [CrossRef]
20. TeGiffel, M.C.; Zwietering, M.H. Validation of predictive models describing the growth of *L. monocytogenes*. *Int. J. Food Microbiol.* **1999**, *46*, 135–149. [CrossRef]
21. Zwietering, M.H.; De Koos, J.T.; Hasenack, B.E.; De Wit, J.C.; Riet, K. Modelling of bacterial growth as a function of temperature. *Appl. Environ. Microbiol.* **1991**, *57*, 1094–1101. [PubMed]
22. Zurera-Cosano, G.; Garciá-Gimeno, R.M.; Rodríguez-Pérez, R.; Hervás-Martínez, C. Performance of response surface model for predition of *L. mesenteroides* growth parameters under different experimental conditions. *Food Control* **2006**, *17*, 429–438. [CrossRef]
23. Baranyi, J.; Pin, C.; Ross, T. Validating and comparing predictive models. *Int. J. Food Microbiol.* **1999**, *48*, 159–166. [CrossRef]
24. Medveďová, A.; Liptáková, D.; Valík, L. Characterization of the growth of *L. rhamnosus* GG in milk at suboptimal temperature. *J. Nutr. Food Res.* **2008**, *47*, 60–67.

25. Medvedova, A.; Mancuskova, T.; Valik, L. Growth of *L. acidophilus* NCFM in dependence on temperature. *Acta Aliment.* **2016**, *45*, 104–111. [CrossRef]
26. Matejčeková, Z.; Liptáková, D.; Spodniaková, S.; Valík, Ľ. Characterisazion of the growth of *L. plantarum* in milk in dependence on temperature. *Acta Chim.* **2016**, *9*, 104–108. [CrossRef]
27. Champagne, C.P.; Gagnon, D.; St. Gelais, D.; Vullemard, J.C. Interactions between *L. lactis* and *S. thermophilus* strains in Cheddar cheese processing conditions. *Int. Dairy J.* **2009**, *19*, 669–674. [CrossRef]
28. Valík, L.; Ačai, P.; Medveďová, A. Application of competitive models in predicting the simultaneous growth of *S. aureus* and lactic acid bacteria in milk. *Food Control* **2018**, *87*, 145–152. [CrossRef]
29. Ačai, P.; Valík, L.; Medveďová, A.; Rosskopf, F. Modelling and predicting the simultaneous growth of *E. coli* and lactic acid bacteria in milk. *Food Sci. Technol. Int.* **2016**, *22*, 475–484. [CrossRef] [PubMed]
30. Šípková, A.; Valík, L.; Liptáková, D.; Pelikánová, J. Effect of lactic acid bacteria on the growth dynamics of *Geotrichum candidum* in fresh cheeses during storage. *J. Food Nutr. Res.* **2014**, *53*, 224–231.
31. Liu, S.Q.; Asmundson, V.; Gopal, P.K.; Holland, R.; Crow, V.L. Influence of reduced water activity on lactose metabolism by *Lactococcus lactis* ssp. *cremoris* at different pH values. *Appl. Environ. Microbiol.* **1998**, *64*, 2111–2116. [PubMed]
32. Woollard, D.C.; Indyk, H.E.; Woollard, G.A. Carnitine in milk: A survey of content, distribution and temporal variation. *Food Chem.* **1999**, *66*, 121–127. [CrossRef]
33. Uguen, P.; Hamelin, J.; Le Pennec, J.P.; Blanco, C. Influence of osmolarity and the presence of an osmoprotectant on *Lactococcus lactis* growth and bacteriocin production. *Appl. Environ. Microbiol.* **1999**, *65*, 291–293.
34. Larsen, R.F.; Añón, M.C. Effect of water activity of milk on acid production by *Streptococcus thermophilus* and *Lactobacillus bulgaricus*. *J. Food Sci.* **1989**, *54*, 917–921. [CrossRef]
35. Ross, T.; Dalgaard, P.; Tienungon, S. Predictive modelling of the growth and survival of *Listeria* in fishery products. *Int. J. Food Microbiol.* **2000**, *62*, 231–246. [CrossRef]
36. Valík, L.; Medveďová, A.; Čižniar, M.; Liptáková, D. Evaluation of temperature effect on growth rate of *Lactobacillus rhamnosus* GG in milk using secondary models. *Chem. Pap.* **2013**, *67*, 737–742. [CrossRef]

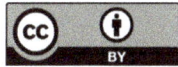

© 2019 by the authors. Licensee MDPI, Basel, Switzerland. This article is an open access article distributed under the terms and conditions of the Creative Commons Attribution (CC BY) license (http://creativecommons.org/licenses/by/4.0/).

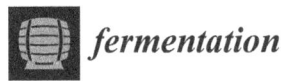

Article

Optimization of Diverse Carbon Sources and Cultivation Conditions for Enhanced Growth and Lipid and Medium-Chain Fatty Acid (MCFA) Production by *Mucor circinelloides*

Syed Ammar Hussain, Yusuf Nazir, Ahsan Hameed, Wu Yang, Kiren Mustafa and Yuanda Song *

Colin Ratledge Center for Microbial Lipids, School of Agriculture Engineering and Food Science, Shandong University of Technology, Zibo 255049, China; ammarshah88@yahoo.com (S.A.H.); yusufnazir91@yahoo.com (Y.N.); ahsanhameed@outlook.com (A.H.); neverhangsome@hotmail.com (W.Y.); mustafakiran92@gmail.com (K.M.)
* Correspondence: ysong@sdut.edu.cn; Tel.: + 86-139-0617-4047

Received: 27 March 2019; Accepted: 18 April 2019; Published: 23 April 2019

Abstract: The effects of various carbon sources and cultivation conditions on the growth kinetics, lipid accumulation, and medium-chain fatty acid (MCFA) production of *Mucor circinelloides* (MC) was investigated for 72 h in shake flask cultivation. Our previous investigation reported increments of 28 to 46% MCFAs among total cell lipids when the MC genome was genetically modified, in comparison to the wild-type. However, the growth of the engineered strain M65-TE-04 was adversely affected. Therefore, the current study was designed to enhance the growth, lipid production, and MCFA productivity of engineered *M. circinelloides* by optimizing the pH, agitation speed, temperature, and carbon sources. The findings for individual variables disclosed that the highest biomass (17.0 g/L) was obtained when coconut oil mixed with glucose was used as a carbon source under normal culture conditions. Additionally, the maximum lipid contents (67.5% cell dry weight (CDW)), MCFA contents (53% total fatty acid (TFA)), and overall lipid productivity (3.53 g/L·d) were attained at 26 °C, pH 6.0, and 150 rpm, respectively. The maximum biomass (19.4 g/L), TFA (14.3g/L), and MCFA (4.71 g/L) contents were achieved with integration of a temperature of 26 °C, pH 6.0, agitation speed 300 rpm, and coconut oil mixed medium as the carbon source. This work illustrates that biomass, TFA, and MCFA contents were increased 1.70–2.0-fold by optimizing the initial pH, agitation speed, temperature, and carbon sources in the *M. circinelloides* engineered strain (M65-TE-04) in comparison to initial cultivation conditions.

Keywords: *Mucor circinelloides*; microbial lipids; medium-chain fatty acids; culture optimization

---

1. Introduction

Currently, single cell oil (SCO) is considered as an alternative and reliable platform to face the challenges related to global warming, scarcity of non-renewable resources, and food security. Over the last decade, medium-chain fatty acids (MCFAs: C8 to C12) and their derivatives have been gaining attention because of their diverse applications in the food, biochemical, and petroleum industries [1]. These MCFAs are involved as precursors in industries involved in the manufacturing of bio-plasticizers, lubricants, detergents, surfactants, adhesives, antibiotics, diverse intermediates for floral fragrances, and flavors [2]. The aforementioned fatty acids have attracted much attraction because they have a positive impact on human health by being easily absorbed and swiftly catabolized through the β-oxidation mechanism, ultimately increasing diet-stimulated thermo-genesis [3]. This mechanism provides a venue for the prevention of various metabolic abnormalities, such as obesity, hyperlipidemia, type II diabetes, atherosclerosis, and cardiovascular diseases (CVDs). The yield of naturally produced

MCFAs from plant (i.e., coconut or palm) sources has been estimated to be insignificant to meet the market demand [2–12]. Therefore, diverse metabolic-engineering strategies have been exploited in different oleaginous microorganisms to augment the contents of MCFAs [13–22]. In addition, numerous investigations have been performed to evaluate the effects of carbon and nitrogen sources, initial pH of the culture medium, C/N ratio, incubation temperature, and their particular effects on the fungal biomass and fatty acid production [23–32]. However, comprehensive information regarding MCFA production under diverse culture conditions is still limited.

Mucor circinelloides is regarded as a model organism for investigations of lipid accumulation. It has been extensively genetically manipulated for the production of diverse biotechnological precursors for the functional food and bio-fuel industries [1,33,34]. However, its fatty acid profile indicates that it is mostly formed by long-chain fatty acids (LCFAs), ultimately making it less attractive for multi-purpose industrial applications. In our previous investigation, efforts to enhance the MCFA content were carried out by integrating different heterologous thioesterase (TE) proteins from plant and bacterial sources into the fatty acid synthase (FAS) complex of the *M. circinelloides* M65 strain, eventually generating mutant strains with significant MCFA-producing capability [1]. Although we successfully enhanced the MCFA contents from the total fatty acids (TFAs), a noteworthy decline in biomass in the resultant strains was observed, which negatively affected the lipid productivity and MCFA contents. Thus, to circumvent the productivity-related challenge stemming from the dry cell weight (CDW) of the *M. circinelloides* strain, M65-TE-04, we synergistically optimized the culture conditions to maximize the yield of MCFAs. The individual and synergistic impact of four key factors, namely the incubation temperature, initial pH, agitation speed, and different carbon sources, were evaluated, and the impact on the biomass and lipid and MCFA contents of *M. circinelloides* strains was elucidated.

2. Material and Methods

2.1. Microorganisms, Culture Conditions, and Experimental Design

The genetically manipulated strain of *M. circinelloides* M65 (i.e., a uracil auxotroph of *M. circinelloides* WJ11), M65-TE-04 (i.e., acyl-ACP-thioesterases: TE-over-expressing strain) from our recent investigation [1], was employed in the present study. This engineered strain was initially inoculated by applying 100 µL of spore suspension (~10^7 spores/mL) into 150 mL of Kendrick and Ratledge (K and R) medium (i.e., 30 g/L glucose, 3.3 g/L ammonium tartrate, 7.0 g/L KH_2PO_4, 2.0 g/L Na_2HPO_4, 1.5 g/L $MgSO_4·7H_2O$, 1.5 g/L yeast extract, 0.1 g/L $CaCl_2·2H_2O$, 8 mg/L $FeCl_3·6H_2O$, 1 mg/L $ZnSO_4·7H_2O$, 0.1 mg/L $CuSO_4·5H_2O$, 0.1 mg/L $Co(NO_3)_2·6H_2O$, and 0.1 mg/L $MnSO_4·5H_2O$ [1] held in a 1 L baffled shake flask. Culture were incubated at 30 °C for 24 h with shaking at 150 rpm and employed at 10% (v/v) to inoculate 1 L baffled shake flask containing 150 mL modified K and R medium (i.e., glucose (80 g/L), coconut oil (30 g/L) with glucose (50 g/L), palm oil (30 g/L) with glucose (50 g/L), glycerol 30 g/L) with glucose (50 g/L), plus essential salts, as mentioned above). To evaluate the effects of the different culture conditions on the growth kinetics and MCFA production, the initial pH, agitation speed, incubation temperature, and different carbon sources were examined using the engineered *M. circinelloides* strain (M65-TE-04). To achieve our aim, a range of pH values (i.e., 4.5, 6.0, 7.5), agitation speeds (i.e., 150 rpm, 220 rpm, 300 rpm), temperatures (i.e., 26 °C, 30 °C, 34 °C), and different carbon sources (i.e., glucose (80 g/L), coconut oil (30 g/L) with glucose (50 g/L), palm oil (30 g/L) with glucose (50 g/L), glycerol 30 g/L) with glucose (50 g/L)) were tested for 72 h in the current investigation. All the materials were autoclaved at 121 °C for 20min. All the above-described chemicals were procured from Millipore Sigma (St. Louis, MO, USA), and all experiments were performed three times for reproducibility purposes.

2.2. Determination of Cell Dry Weight (CDW)

Harvesting of the fungal biomass was carried out according to our previously described method [1]. In brief, a suction filtration method was employed followed by three washes with double-distilled water to eliminate possible medium contents. The collected samples were then frozen at −80 °C overnight, and the samples were lyophilized for 24 h. The fungal biomass weight was calculated by the gravimetrical method.

The biomass productivity (P_{DCW}) of fungal cells was computed using the following equation:

$$P_{DCW} \text{ (g/L·d)} = (CDW_f - CDW_i)/(T_f - T_i) \quad (1)$$

2.3. Total Lipid and Fatty Acid Profiling

Lipid extraction was performed according to a previously developed method with minor modifications [1]. In brief, 20 mg of lyophilized biomass was mixed with chloroform/methanol (2:1, v/v). Methylation was carried out with 10% (v/v) methanolic HCl at 60 °C for 4 h. Pentadecanoic acid (15:0) (Millipore Sigma, St. Louis, MO, USA) was used as an internal standard for the lyophilized cells before methylation. Finally, the fatty acid methyl esters (FAMEs) were extracted with n-hexane and subsequently analyzed by GC using the DB-Waxetr column with the following specifications: film thickness 0.25 μm, 30 m×0.32 mm (Shimadzu Co., Ltd., Kyoto, Japan). The program used for the gas chromatography (GC) was as follows: 120 °C for 3 min, ramp to 200 °C at 5 °C min^{-1}, ramp to 220 °C at 4 °C min^{-1}, and hold for 2 min [1,33].

Lipid productivity (P_{Lipid}) and MCFA productivity (P_{MCFA}) were calculated as follows:

$$P_{Lipid} \text{ (g/L·d)} = (Lipid_f - Lipid_i)/(T_f - T_i) \quad (2)$$

$$P_{MCFA} \text{ (g/L·d)} = (MCFA_f - MCFA_i)/(T_f - T_i) \quad (3)$$

where C_f is the final lipid content (g/L), C_i is initial lipid content, and TL is the total lipid content.

2.4. Construction of Orthogonal Matrix Design (OMD)

The synergistic effect of all parameters was evaluated on the bases of OMD design, as shown in Table 1.

Table 1. Orthogonal matrix design (OMD) to evaluate the diverse culture conditions (coded values for factors and their levels).

Factors	Code 1	Code 2	Code 3	Code 4
Temperature	24 °C	26 °C	30 °C	34 °C
Agitation	150rpm	220rpm	300rpm	–
pH	4.5	6	7.5	–
Carbon Source	Glucose	Palm-oil + glucose	Coconut-oil + glucose	Glycerol + glucose

2.5. Statistical Analysis

A statistical analysis of the acquired data was performed with SPSS 16.0 for Windows (SPSS Inc., Chicago, IL, USA). Mean values and the standard error of the mean were computed from the data gathered from three independent experiments. The Student's t-test was employed to estimate differences between the data, and $p < 0.05$ was regarded as a significant difference.

3. Results and Discussion

To investigate the effect of diverse cultivation conditions of the *M. circinelloides* strain (i.e., M65-TE-04) on cell growth, lipid accumulation, and MCFA production, four key cultivation factors (i.e., incubation temperature, initial pH, speed of agitation, and carbon-sources) were assessed in a first stage individually, and in a second stage in a combinatorial study following orthogonal matrix design (OMD). When individual culture conditions were evaluated, all the remaining culture factors were held constant. These conditions were analogous to the normal culture conditions to eventually attain particular conclusions on the basis of relevant variable effects on cell growth and lipid accumulation.

3.1. Effect of Incubation Temperature on Fungal Biomass and Lipid Accumulation

Fungal biomass, lipid accumulation, and MCFA contents of *M. circinelloides* strain M65-TE-04 cultured on modified K and R medium were appraised at three different temperatures (i.e., 26 °C, 30 °C, and 34 °C) for 72 h. After 3 days of cultivation, the biomass (CDW, g/L) acquired at the different temperatures is shown in Figure 1A. Overall, we noticed a fluctuation of fungal growth at different cultivation temperatures. The biomass at 26 °C was considerably higher (i.e., 13 g/L) than at other temperatures. The quantity of biomass gradually declined with an increase in temperature (i.e., 9.5 g/L and 4.6 g/L for 30 °C and 34 °C, respectively) (Figure 1A). This pattern clearly demonstrated that higher temperature was not appropriate for fungal cell growth.

Temperature is regarded as a crucial factor for fungal cell growth, overall lipid productivity, and specifically MCFA contents. We noticed an inverse correlation between the cultivation temperature and MCFA contents. High MCFA contents were found at 26 °C (i.e., 50%), which were approximately 1.3-fold higher than the titer obtained at 34 °C (Figure 1A). Likewise, the lipid contents (% CDW) also declined with the temperature elevation (Figure 1B). The maximum lipid accumulation was obtained at 26 °C, which was almost 63% higher than that at 34 °C. Finally, we noticed a considerable fluctuation in biomass and lipid productivity ($p > 0.05$), as shown in Figure 1C. These outcomes indicated that the optimal temperature for fungal cell growth, as well as for lipid and MCFA productivity, was 26 °C. The maximum biomass (i.e., 4.37 g/L·d) and lipid productivity (i.e., 2.93 g/L·d) were achieved at 26 °C. Our results are in agreement with a previous investigation conducted using *M. circinelloides* strains, which demonstrated maximum cell growth and lipid production at temperatures ranging from 26 °C to 30 °C [34,35]. Moreover, the optimum temperature for growth and lipid accumulation in other fungal strain has been estimated to range from 26 °C to 30 °C [36].

3.2. Effect of the Initial pH of the Culture Medium on Fungal Biomass and Lipid Accumulation

In the current investigation, the *M. circinelloides* strain (i.e., M65-TE-04) was able to grow at different pH values (i.e., 4.5, 6.0, and 7.5) (Figure 2A). Overall, pH values below or above 6.0 had drastic effects on the growth of *M. circinelloides* strains, as growth declined after 24 h of the cultivation period. Although *M. circinelloides* strains could grow within a wide pH range, the maximum growth was observed at pH 6.0. The highest biomass content (CDW; 12.5 ± 2.1 g/L) was achieved in culture at an initial pH of 6.0 over culture duration of 72 h. The biomass of *M. circinelloides* strains at different pH values is elaborated in Figure 2A. Our findings are in agreement with our previous studies [1]. However, some authors have reported that the fungal growth rate was found to be maximal at pH 4.5 [37].

The pH value is a crucial cultivation factor that affects cell surface characteristics, ultimately modifying the cellular permeability capacity for different ions, bases, and acids across the membrane. It also has a great influence on the cellular metabolism of carbohydrates, proteins, and lipids. Moreover, the depletion of nutrients, i.e., phosphorus, nitrogen, or sulfur, also affects biochemical processes in the microorganism. Thus, in the current investigation, we provided an altered nutrient supply to fungal strain by using the different initial pHs of culture mediums (i.e., 4.5, 6.0, and 7.5). As depicted in Figure 2B, we observed that increasing the pH (4.5 to 6.0) had a positive effect on the TFA content (% CDW). More precisely, the maximum lipid contents were obtained at pH 6.0 (i.e., 64.3% of CDW). Similarly, the MCFA contents were slightly influenced by the initial culture pH, and maximum MCFA contents (% CDW) were attained at pH 6.0 (Figure 2A). However, no obvious alterations in other saturated fatty acids were observed for all culture initial pH values. There were no significant changes in lipid and MCFA contents at pH 4.5 and 7.5 (Figure 2A,B).

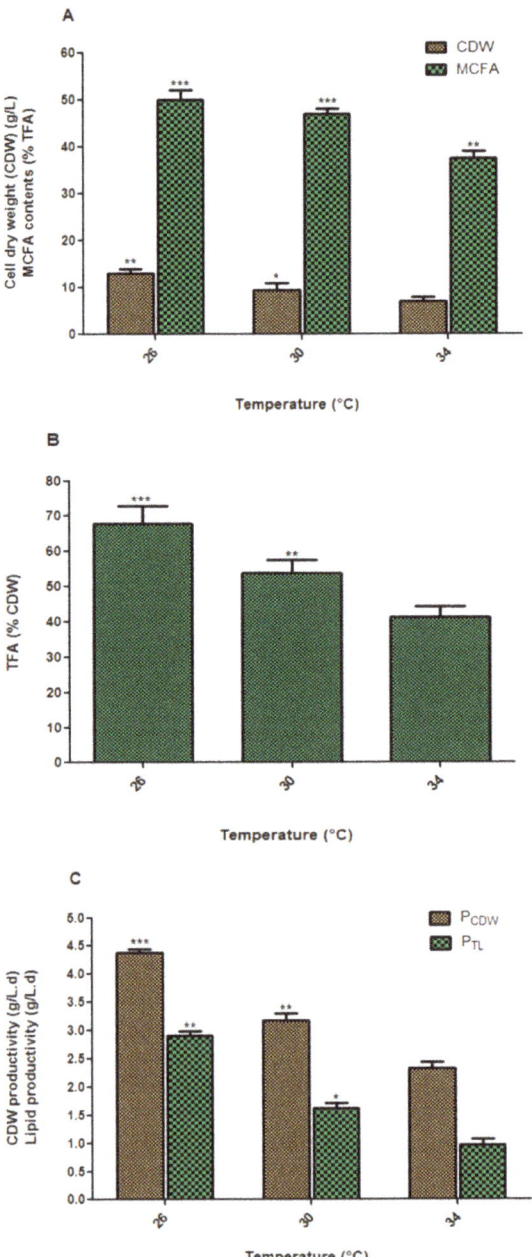

Figure 1. (**A**–**C**) Effect of temperature on (**A**) cell dry weight (CDW, g/L) and MCFA content (% TLC), (**B**) fungal TFA (% CDW), (**C**) biomass productivity (P_{CDW}, g/L·d), and lipid productivity (P_{TL}, g/L·d) of the *M. circinelloides* strain (i.e., M65-TE-04) after 72 h (3 days) of cultivation. Values are the mean of three independent experiments. Error bars show the standard error of the mean. Asterisks indicate that the differences (* $p < 0.05$; ** $p < 0.01$; *** $p < 0.001$) between the means of different treatments are statistically significant.

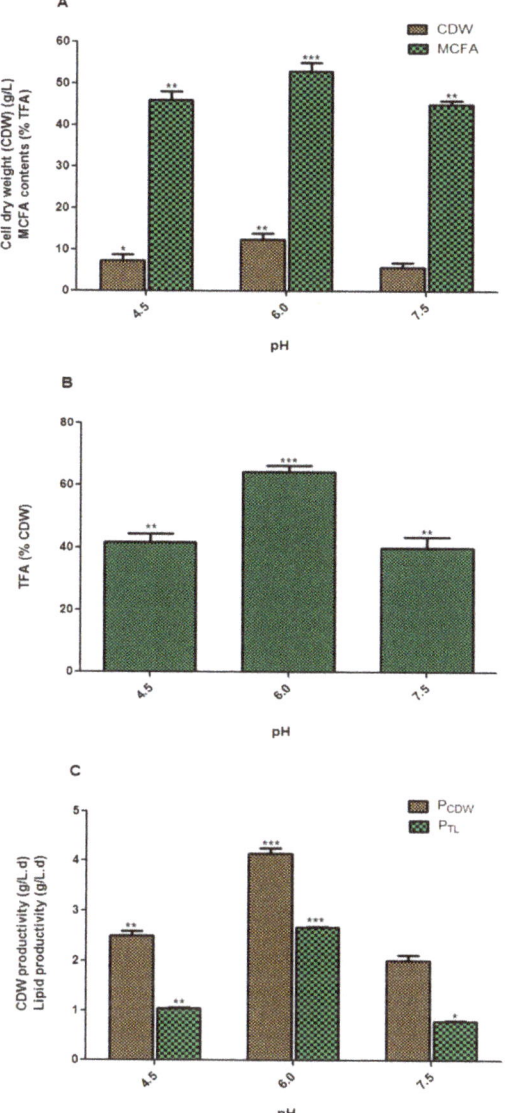

Figure 2. (**A–C**) Effect of initial pH on (**A**) cell dry weight (CDW, g/L) and MCFA content (% TLC), (**B**) fungal TFA (% CDW), (**C**) biomass productivity (P_{CDW}, g/L·d), and lipid productivity (P_{TL}, g/L·d) of the *M. circinelloides* strain (i.e., M65-TE-04) after 72 h (3 days) of cultivation. Values are the mean of three independent experiments. Error bars show the standard error of the mean. Asterisks indicate that the differences (* $p < 0.05$; ** $p < 0.01$; *** $p < 0.001$) between the means of different treatments are statistically significant.

The association of cell dry weight (CDW) and lipid productivities (g/L) provided noteworthy insight into cell growth at different initial pH values of the culture medium. The biomass and lipid productivities are mentioned in Figure 2C. The maximum biomass and lipid productivity were achieved at pH 6.0, whereas the minimum productivities for the biomass and lipid contents were found at pH 7.5 (Figure 2C). A previous report has shown that the pH values of fungal cells are sustained by ion exchange systems across the cell membranes, which eventually fabricate the electric potential with an intracellular positive charge at the cost of cellular energy. At a pH value other than the optimal level for fungal biomass growth, more energy is required to properly maintain the physiological tasks. Therefore, biomass and lipid productivities are maximal at pH 6.0 [33,34,38].

3.3. Effect of Agitation Speed on Fungal Biomass and Lipid Accumulation

When all the culture parameters (i.e., substrate, temperature, initial pH, etc.) of the culture medium were optimized, the specific growth rate was solely associated with the accessibility of dissolved oxygen (DO). To improve the DO, we cultured fungal strain M64-TE-04 at diverse agitation speeds (i.e., 150, 220, and 300 rpm). The fungal biomass, lipid accumulation, and MCFA contents and their productivities are demonstrated in Figure 3A–C. We observed a significant change in biomass and MCFA contents with a corresponding increase in agitation speed from 150 to 220 rpm (Figure 3A). Moreover, a noteworthy difference in total lipid contents was noticed at an agitation speed of 220 rpm (Figure 3B). Overall, the biomass and lipid productivities increased from 150 to 220 rpm and then decreased from 220 to 300 rpm (Figure 3C). It has been previously reported that cells grow and multiply more rapidly to the optimum level in the presence of a high oxygen compared with a low oxygen supply, ultimately enhancing the biomass and lipid productivities [39,40]. The specific growth rate demonstrated an increment from 150 to 220 rpm (i.e., 2.1 d^{-1} to 3.5 d^{-1}). Conversely, increases in agitation speed above 220 rpm negatively affected the growth rate to 1.55 d^{-1}. The *M. circinelloides* strains were susceptible to a high agitation speed, and the overall growth rate declined above 300 rpm [41].

3.4. Effect of Carbon Sources on Fungal Biomass and Lipid Accumulation

Among the essential nutrients, carbon source plays a promising role in the fermentation process because carbon sources are directly correlated with the fungal biomass and cellular metabolites. To evaluate an appropriate carbon source for optimum fungal cell growth, total lipid productivity, and MCFA production, three different carbon sources were employed as additional carbon sources along with modified K and R medium. A previous investigation has shown that coconut oil, palm oil, and some other vegetable oils (i.e., mostly consist of lauric acid, myristic acid, and palmitic acid) containing culture medium show positive effects on fungal biomass and lipid accumulation [42]. Thus, to elucidate the effects of the aforementioned oils on MCFAs, we cultured the engineered strain M65-TE-04 in modified K and R medium together with coconut oil (3%), palm oil (3%), glycerol (3%), or sole glucose (for the control experiments). We chose these concentrations based on some of our preliminary work (data not shown), as well as our previous investigation using 3% diverse oils [43]. The cell dry weight (CDW) and TFA contents for strain M65-TE-04 were shown in Figure 4A,B. The aforementioned fungal strains showed a maximum CDW with coconut oil mixed medium, i.e., 17.0 g/L at 72 h of the cultivation period. The CDW for palm oil mixed medium and medium containing glycerol as a supplement were 13.0 g/L and 10.0 g/L, respectively, which is appreciably higher in comparison to fungal cell cultured in only glucose-containing medium (9.0 g/L) (Figure 4A). The TFA contents (% CDW) were found to be 9.5% higher when the fungal strain M65-TE-04 was cultured in coconut oil mixed medium in comparison to control (Figure 4B). Interestingly, the highest CDW was determined for strain M65-TE-04 grown in coconut oil mixed medium over 72 h. However, the highest TFA content in the aforementioned strain was obtained when the cells were grown in coconut oil.

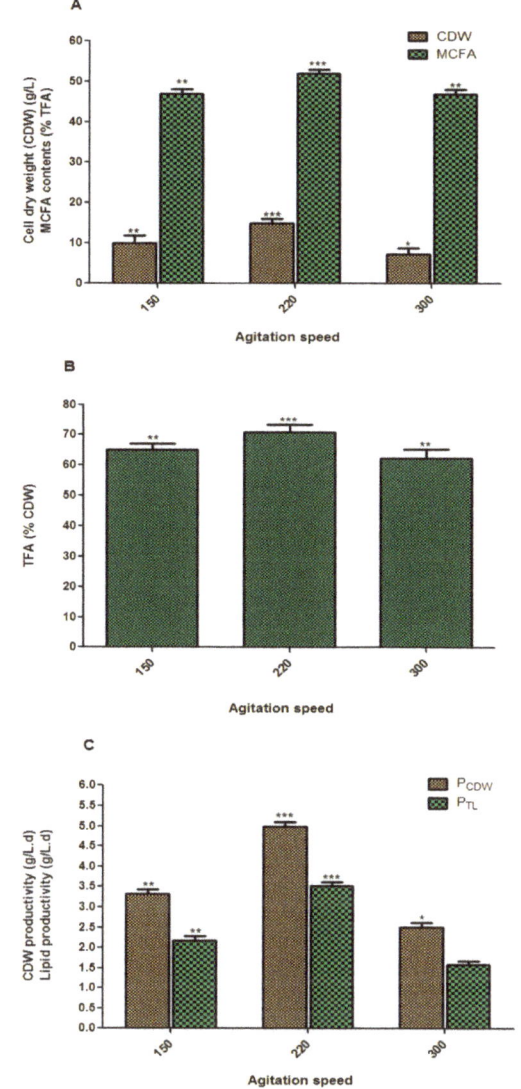

Figure 3. (**A–C**) Effect of agitation speed on (**A**) cell dry weight (CDW, g/L) and MCFA content (% TLC), (**B**) fungal TFA (% CDW), (**C**) biomass productivity (P_{CDW}, g/L·d), and lipid productivity (P_{TL}, g/L·d) of the *M. circinelloides* strain (i.e., M65-TE-04) after 72 h (3 days) of cultivation. Values are the mean of three independent experiments. Error bars show the standard error of the mean. Asterisks indicate that the differences (* $p < 0.05$; ** $p < 0.01$; *** $p < 0.001$) between the means of different treatments are statistically significant.

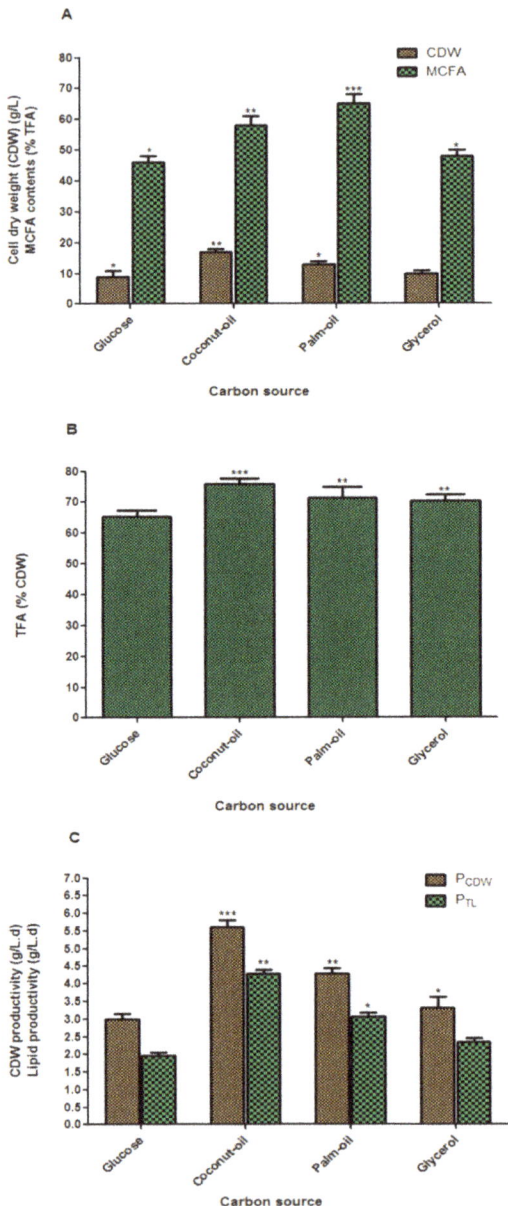

Figure 4. (**A–C**) Effect of different carbon sources on (**A**) cell dry weight (CDW, g/L) and MCFA content (% TLC), (**B**) fungal TFA (% CDW), (**C**) biomass productivity (P_{CDW}, g/L·d), and lipid productivity (P_{TL}, g/L·d) of the *M. circinelloides* strain (i.e., M65-TE-04) after 72 h (3 days) of cultivation. Values are the mean of three independent experiments. Error bars show the standard error of the mean. Asterisks indicate that the differences (* $p < 0.05$; ** $p < 0.01$; *** $p < 0.001$) between the means of different treatments are statistically significant.

The majority of the fatty acids in the *M. circinelloides* strain were palmitic acid, stearic acid, oleic acid, linoleic acid, and γ-linolenicacid. We observed a noteworthy difference in the fatty acid profile when strain M65-TE-04 was cultured in diverse glucose oil mixed medium. The fatty acid profile of *M. circinelloides* strain M65-TE-04 was directly associated with the fatty acid compositions of the glucose oil medium (Figure 5). The highest MCFA contents (i.e., 65% CDW) were obtained when the fungal cells were grown in medium containing palm oil as a supplement (Figure 4A). In contrast, significant outcomes related to TFA contents were obtained when the fungal strain was grown in coconut oil mixed medium (Figure 4B). The biomass and lipid productivities ($p > 0.05$) for culture media containing different carbon sources are shown in Figure 4C.

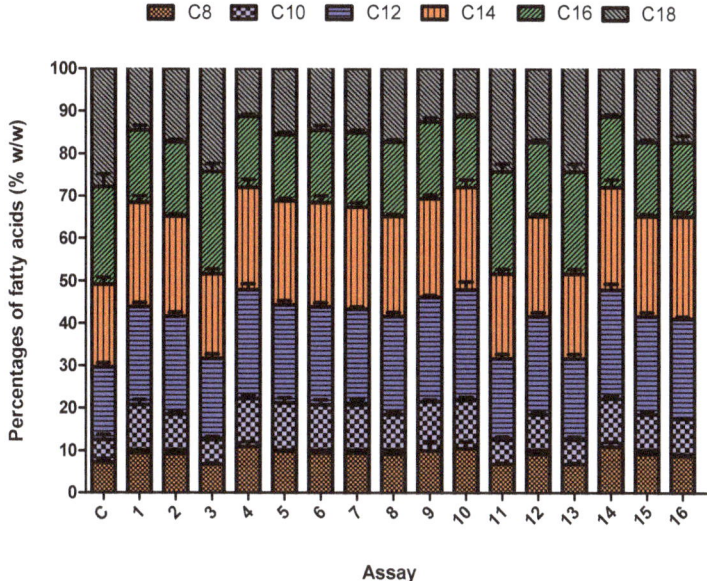

Figure 5. Fatty acid profile (% of TFA) of the *M. circinelloides* strain (i.e., M65-TE-04) in the presence of differences in pH, agitation speed, temperature, and carbon sources based on the orthogonal matrix design (OMD). The samples were harvested after 72 h (3 days) of cultivation. Values are the mean of three independent experiments. Error bars show the standard error of the mean.

Our results are consistent with previous studies showing that fungal cells produce more fungal biomass and total lipids when grown in medium-chain-containing oils [42–44]. Based on our results, the highest biomass and lipid productivities were achieved with coconut oil mixed medium (g/L·d), while the maximum MCFA contents in terms of the percentage of CDW were obtained with palm oil mixed medium (Figure 4C).

Taken together, we acquired diverse results among all individual variables for the culture growth conditions. Likewise, the highest biomass was obtained when coconut oil mixed medium was used as a carbon source under normal culture conditions; additionally, the highest fatty acid contents (% CDW) were achieved at 26 °C, the highest MCFA contents (% CDW) with palm oil mixed medium, and the maximum overall lipid productivity (8.6 g/L·d) with coconut oil supplementation. Since we obtained diverse outcomes under the different culture conditions, synergetic insights into the individual culture conditions are needed to evaluate the different combinations based on an orthogonal matrix design (OMD).

3.5. Synergistic Effect of the Culture Conditions on Fungal Biomass and Lipid Accumulation

To investigate cell growth and lipid accumulation of the strain *M. circinelloides* M65-TE-04, the fungal cells were cultured under different conditions. The coded values of individual variables by the orthogonal matrix design (OMD) are provided in Table 1. All the experiments were carried out in a 1-L baffled shake flask with 250 mL modified K and R medium containing glucose or other carbon sources (see Section 2.1 for details). The responses for the four independent variables (i.e., temperature, agitation, pH, and carbon sources) obtained based on the orthogonal matrix design (OMD) (SPSS 19) were provided in Table 2.

Table 2. Orthogonal matrix design (OMD) for the combination of different culture conditions (coded values) and their responses in biomass contents (CDW, g/L), lipid contents (TFA,% CDW), MCFA contents (MCFA,% TFA), lipid productivity (P_{TL}, mg/L·d), and MCFA productivity (P_{MCFA}, mg/L·d) of *M. circinelloides* strain (i.e., M65-TE-04) after 72 h (3 days) of cultivation period. Values were the mean of three independent experiments.

Assay	pH	Agitation speed	Temperature	Carbon-Source	CDW	TFA	MCFA	C_{TL}	C_{MCFA}	P_{TL}	P_{MCFA}	Yield
1	1	1	1	1	6.4	45.5	44.72	2.9	1.3	967	435	0.016
2	3	3	1	3	3.3	55.45	48.25	1.8	0.86	600	286	0.010
3	1	1	1	4	4.3	32.2	32.48	1.3	0.42	434	140	0.005
4	2	2	1	2	10.7	69.2	55.25	7.4	4.01	2467	1337	0.051
5	2	1	3	1	8.2	56.7	46.45	4.6	2.1	1534	700	0.026
6	1	3	2	1	4.5	26.7	39.25	1.7	0.66	567	220	0.008
7	3	2	4	1	7.8	18.2	52.3	1.4	0.73	467	244	0.009
8	1	1	4	3	5.4	13.5	35.23	0.72	0.25	240	84	0.003
9	1	1	4	2	4.5	16.9	45.26	0.76	0.34	254	114	0.004
10	1	3	3	2	6.5	22.5	40.29	1.4	1.61	467	538	0.020
11	2	3	4	4	9.7	40.3	42.49	3.9	1.65	1300	550	0.020
12	2	1	2	3	16.3	67.1	49.47	10.1	5.01	3368	1670	0.062
13	3	1	3	4	8.8	30.45	42.29	2.6	1.1	867	367	0.013
14	3	1	2	2	11.5	38.22	39.21	4.39	1.7	1464	569	0.021
15	1	2	3	3	3.6	36.2	48.45	1.3	0.62	434	207	0.007
16	2	3	2	3	19.4	74.1	54.2	14.3	4.71	4767	2570	0.058

C_{TL}: lipid content (g/L); C_{MCFA}: MCFA content (g/L); P_{TL}: lipid productivity (mg/L·d); P_{MCFA}: MCFA productivity (mg/L·d).

We observed an elevation in biomass in assays 12 and 16 and a slight elevation in assays 14 and 4, while the lipid contents (% CDW) exceeded the maximum in assay 16 and significantly exceeded the maximum in assays 12 and 4. Assays 2 and 5 also showed higher lipid contents (% CDW). Overall, assays 16, 12, and 4 demonstrated the highest lipid (g/L) and MCFA contents (g/L), as well as lipid and MCFA productivities (mg/L·d), as shown in Table 2. Thus, from the above discussion and the results represented in Table 2, we concluded that assay 16 with specific cultivation conditions (i.e., temperature 26 °C, pH 6, agitation speed 300 rpm, 3% coconut oil mixed medium as the carbon source) provided the best outcome for *M. circinelloides* strain M65-TE-04among all 16 assays. This condition eventually provided the highest lipid (i.e., 4767 mg/L·d) and MCFA productivity (i.e., 2570 mg/L·d) (Table 2). The higher contents of MCFA obtained in *M. circinelloides* (M65-TE-04) by using coconut oil. This is might be due to availability of MCFA in coconut oil, and therefore it shows that *M. circinelloides* should assimilate the MCFA from the coconut into their cells.

M. circinelloides naturally produces LCFAs, eventually making it less attractive for use as a precursor in the food, biochemical, and aviation industries. In our recent investigation, we genetically manipulated *M. circinelloides* strain M65, ultimately to obtain mutant strains with high MCFA-producing ability. Although we were successful, the resultant strains showed a very low biomass, which eventually affected the lipid and MCFA productivity [1]. Thus, the approach used in the present study, optimizing the cultivation conditions (i.e., assay 16) to enhance the MCFA yield (g/L) and contents (% TFA) in *M. circinelloides*, fulfilled the primary objective of the current investigation. No studies have yet been conducted in this respect. The utilization of different agriculture by-products (i.e., copra cake, palm fruit cake) as supplementation for the culture medium, which would be environmentally friendly and cost effective, is our next possible objective.

4. Conclusions

In the current investigation, we assessed whether the capability of the engineered strain of *M. circinelloides* (i.e., M65-TE-04) to generate MCFAs could be improved by choosing appropriate culture medium ingredients and culture conditions. We noticed significant increments (%) in biomass, TFA, and MCFA contents (i.e., 112.25%, 139.93%, and 70% respectively) by applying the combination of physical parameters: temperature 26 °C, pH 6, agitation speed 300 rpm, and 3% coconut oil mixed medium as the carbon source. These results suggested that *M. circinelloides* strain M65-TE-04 could utilize a common lipid to overproduce MCFAs, thus revealing the extensive biotechnological significance of this fungus. The coconut oil mixed medium stimulated fungal cell growth and MCFA production more effectively than palm oil and glycerol. However, sufficient space remains to enhance MCFA production in *M. circinelloides* through the use of diverse strategies. Conclusively, this investigation could be used to further exploit industrial MCFA production using the engineered *M. circinelloides* strain.

Author Contributions: S.A.H. and Y.N. carried out the experiments. S.A.H. drafted the manuscript. A.H., W.Y., and K.M. assisted in GC analysis. Y.S. conceived the study, participated in the experimental design, and reviewed the final manuscript. All authors read and approved the final manuscript.

Funding: This work was supported by National Natural Science Foundation of China (31670064), TaiShan Industrial Experts Program (tscy 20160101), Chinese Government Scholarship Council (CSC), and starting grant from Shandong University of Technology.

Acknowledgments: We thank to Wu Yang for technical support. We are also indebted to Scarlett Geunes-Boyer and Alexis Garcia for critical reading and discussions.

Conflicts of Interest: The authors declare no competing interests.

References

1. Hussain, S.A.; Hameed, A.; Khan, M.A.K.; Zhang, Y.; Zhang, H.; Garre, V.; Song, Y. Engineering of Fatty Acid Synthases (FASs) to Boost the Production of Medium-Chain Fatty Acids (MCFAs) in *Mucor circinelloides*. *Int. J. Mol. Sci.* **2019**, *20*, 786. [CrossRef] [PubMed]
2. Sarria, S.; Kruyer, N.S.; Yahya, P.P. Microbial synthesis of medium-chain chemicals from renewable. *Nat. Biotechnol.* **2017**, *35*, 1158–1166. [CrossRef] [PubMed]
3. Nagao, K.; Yanagita, T. Medium-chain fatty acids: Functional lipids for the prevention and treatment of the metabolic syndrome. *Pharm. Res.* **2010**, *61*, 208–212. [CrossRef]
4. Torella, J.P.; Ford, T.J.; Kim, S.N.; Chen, A.M.; Way, J.C.; Silver, P.A. Tailored fatty acid synthesis via dynamic control of fatty acid elongation. *Proc. Nat. Acad. Sci. USA.* **2013**, *110*, 11290–11295. [CrossRef] [PubMed]
5. Leber, C.; Da-Silva, N.A. Engineering of *Saccharomyces cerevisiae* for the synthesis of short chain fatty acids. *Biotechnol. Bioeng.* **2014**, *111*, 347–358. [CrossRef] [PubMed]
6. Xu, P.; Qiao, K.; Ahn, W.S. Stephanopoulos, G. Engineering *Yarrowia lipolytica* as a platform for synthesis of drop-in transportation fuels and oleochemicals. *Proc. Natl. Acad. Sci. USA.* **2016**, *113*, 10848–10853. [CrossRef]
7. Zhu, Z.; Zhou, Y.J.; Krivoruchko, A.; Grininger, M.; Zhao, Z.K.; Nielsen, J. Expanding the product portfolio of fungal type I fatty acid synthases. *Nat. Chem. Biol.* **2017**, *13*, 360–362. [CrossRef] [PubMed]
8. Liu, X.; Hicks, W.M.; Silver, P.A.; Way, J.C. Engineering acyl carrier protein to enhance production of shortened fatty acids. *Biotechnol. Biofuel* **2016**, *9*, 24. [CrossRef] [PubMed]
9. Gajewski, J.; Pavlovic, R.; Fischer, M.; Boles, E.; Grininger, M. Engineering fungal de novo fatty acid synthesis for short chain fatty acid production. *Nat. Commun.* **2017**, *8*, 14650. [CrossRef]
10. Liu, H.; Cheng, T.; Xian, M.; Cao, Y.; Fang, F.; Zou, H. Fatty acid from the renewable sources: A promising feedstock for the production of biofuels and biobased chemicals. *Biotechnol. Adv.* **2014**, *32*, 382–389. [CrossRef] [PubMed]
11. Lynd, L.R.; Zyl, V.W.H.; Mc Bride, J.E.; Laser, M. Consolidated bioprocessing of cellulosic biomass: An update. *Curr. Opin. Biotechnol.* **2005**, *16*, 577–583. [CrossRef] [PubMed]
12. Runguphan, W.; Keasling, J.D. Metabolic engineering of Saccharomyces cerevisiae for production of fatty acid-derived biofuels and chemicals. *Metab. Eng.* **2014**, *21*, 103–113. [CrossRef] [PubMed]

13. Lian, J.; Zhao, H. Reversal of the β-oxidation cycle in *Saccharomyces cerevisiae* for production of fuels and chemicals. *ACS Synth. Biol.* **2015**, *4*, 332–341. [CrossRef]
14. Dellomonaco, C.; Clomburg, J.M.; Miller, E.N.; Gonzalez, R. Engineered reversal of the β-oxidation cycle for the synthesis of fuels and chemicals. *Nature* **2011**, *476*, 355–3559. [CrossRef] [PubMed]
15. Kim, S.; Clomburg, J.M.; Gonzalez, R. Synthesis of medium-chain length (C6-C10) fuels and chemicals via β-oxidation reversal in *Escherichia coli*. *J. Ind. Microbiol. Biotechnol.* **2015**, *42*, 465–475. [CrossRef] [PubMed]
16. Grisewood, M.J.; Grisewood, M.J.; Hernandez Lozada, N.J.; Thoden, J.B.; Gifford, N.P.; Mendez-Perez, D.; Schoenberger, H.A.; Allan, M.F.; Floy, M.E.; Lai, R.Y.; Holden, H.M.; et al. Computational redesign of acyl-ACP thioesterase with improved selectivity toward medium-chain-length fatty acids. *ACS Catal.* **2017**, *7*, 3837–3849. [CrossRef] [PubMed]
17. Ageitos, J.M.; Vallejo, J.A.; Veiga-Crespo, P.; Villa, T.G. Oily yeasts as oleaginous cell factories. *Appl. Microbiol. Biotechnol.* **2011**, *90*, 1219–1227. [CrossRef]
18. Beopoulos, A.; Chardo, T.; Nicaud, J.M. *Yarrowia lipolytica*: A model and a tool to understand the mechanisms implicated in lipid accumulation. *Biochimie* **2009**, *91*, 692–696. [CrossRef]
19. Papanikolaou, S.; Aggelis, G. Lipids of oleaginous yeasts. Part II: Technology and potential applications. *Euro. J. Lipid Sci. Technol.* **2011**, *113*, 1052–1073. [CrossRef]
20. Huan, L.; Zhao, L.; Zan, X.; Song, Y.; Ratledge, C. Boosting fatty acid synthesis in *Rhodococcus opacus* PD630 by overexpression of autologous thioesterases. *Biotechnol. Lett.* **2016**, *38*, 999–1008. [CrossRef]
21. Rigouin, C.; Croux, C.; Borsenberger, V.; Khaled, M.B.; Chardot, T.; Marty, A.; Bordes, F. Increasing medium chain fatty acids production in *Yarrowia lipolytica* by metabolic engineering. *Microb. Cell Fact.* **2018**, *17*, 142. [CrossRef] [PubMed]
22. Chen, L.; Zhang, J.; Chen, W.N. Engineering the *Saccharomyces cerevisiae* β-Oxidation Pathway to Increase Medium Chain Fatty Acid Production as Potential Biofuel. *PLoS ONE* **2014**, *9*, e84853. [CrossRef] [PubMed]
23. Aggelis, G. Two alternative pathways for substrate assimilation by *Mucor circinelloides*. *Folia Microbiol.* **1996**, *41*, 254–256. [CrossRef]
24. Chen, H.C.; Liu, T.M. Inoculum effects on the production of γ-linolenic acid by the shake culture of *Cunninghamella echinulata* CCRC 31840. *Enz. Microb. Technol.* **1997**, *21*, 137–142. [CrossRef]
25. Conti, E.; Stredansky, M.; Stredanska, S.; Zanetti, F. γ-Linolenic acid production by solid-state fermentation of Mucorales strains on cereals. *Bioresour. Technol.* **2001**, *76*, 283–286. [CrossRef]
26. Emelyanova, E.V. Lipid and γ-linolenic acid production by *Mucor inaquisporus*. *Proc. Biochem.* **1997**, *32*, 173–177. [CrossRef]
27. Roux, M.P.; Kock, J.L.F.; Du Preez, J.C.; Botha, A. The influence of dissolved oxygen tension on the production of cocoa butter equivalents and gamma-linolenic acid by *Mucor circinelloides*. *System. Appl. Microbiol.* **1995**, *18*, 329–334. [CrossRef]
28. Khan, M.A.K.; Yang, J.; Hussain, S.A.; Zhang, H.; Garre, V.; Song, Y. Genetic modification of *Mucor circinelloides* to construct stearidonic acid producing cell factory. *Int. J. Mol. Sci.* **2019**, *20*, 1683. [CrossRef]
29. Stredansky, M.; Conti, E.; Stredanska, S.; Zanetti, F. γ-linolenic acid production with *Thamnidium elegans* by solid state fermentation on apple pomace. *Bioresour. Technol.* **2000**, *73*, 41–45. [CrossRef]
30. Tauk-Tornisielo, S.M.; Vieira, J.M.; Carneiro, M.C.V.S.; Govone, J.S. Fatty acid production by four strains of *Mucor hiemalis* grown in plant oil and soluble carbohydrates. *Afr. J. Biotechnol.* **2007**, *6*, 1840–1847.
31. Torlanova, B.O.; Funtikova, N.S.; Konova, I.V.; Babanova, N.K. Synthesis of the lipid complex containing gamma-linolenic acid and carotenoids by a mucorous fungus under various cultivation conditions. *Microbiology* **1995**, *64*, 492–496.
32. Vaughn, D.M.; Reinhart, G.A. Influence dietary fatty acid ratios on tissue eicosanoid production and blood coagulation parameters in dog. In *Recent Advances in Canine and Feline Nutritional Research—Ians International Nutrition Symposium*; Orange Frazer Press: Wilmington, OH, USA, 1996; pp. 243–255.
33. Khan, M.A.K.; Yang, J.; Luan, X.; Hussain, S.A.; Zhang, H.; Liang, L.; Garre, V.; Song, Y. Construction of DGLA producing cell factory by genetic modification of *Mucor circinelloides*. *Microb. Cell Fact.* **2019**, *18*, 64. [CrossRef] [PubMed]
34. Xia, C.; Zhang, J.; Zhang, W.; Hu, B. A new cultivation method for microbial oil production: cell pelletization and lipid accumulation by *Mucor circinelloides*. *Biotechnol. Biofuels* **2011**, *4*, 15. [CrossRef]
35. Morin-Sardin, S.K.; Coroller, L.; Jany, J.L.; Coton, E. Effect of temperature, pH, and water activity on Mucor spp. growth on synthetic medium, cheese analog and cheese. *Food Microbiol.* **2016**, *56*, 69–79. [PubMed]

36. Suutari, M. Effect of growth temperature on lipid fatty acids of four fungi (*Aspergillus niger, Nurosporacrassa, Penicillium chrysogenum* and *Trichoderma reesei*. *Arc. Micro.* **1995**, *164*, 212–216. [CrossRef]
37. Vylkova, S. Environmental pH modulation by pathogenic fungi as a strategy to conquer the host. *PLoS Pathog.* **2017**, *13*, e1006149. [CrossRef] [PubMed]
38. Trzaska, W.J.; Correia, J.N.; Villegas, M.T.; May, R.C.; Voelz, K. pH Manipulation as a Novel Strategy for Treating Mucormycosis. *Anti Age. Chemother.* **2015**, *59*, 6968–6974. [CrossRef] [PubMed]
39. Azmi, W.; Thakur, M.; Javed, A.; Thakur, N. Interactive Effect of Agitation Speed and Aeration Rate on Heat Stable β-carotene Production From *Mucor azygosporus* Using Deprotenized Waste Whey Filtrate in Stirred Tank Reactor. *Curr. Biochem. Engin.* **2015**, *2*, 65–72. [CrossRef]
40. Ibrahim, D.; Weloosamy, H.; Lim, S.H. Effect of agitation speed on the morphology of *Aspergillus niger* HFD5A-1 hyphae and its pectinase production in submerged fermentation. *World J. Biol. Chem.* **2015**, *6*, 265–271. [CrossRef]
41. Saad, N.; Abdeshahian, P.; Kalil, M.S.; Yusoff, W.M.W.; Hamid, A.A. Optimization of Aeration and Agitation Rate for Lipid and Gamma Linolenic Acid Productio by *Cunningha mellabainieri* 2A1 in Submerged Fermentation Using Response Surface Methodology. *Sci. World J.* **2014**, *2014*, 280146. [CrossRef]
42. Zan, X.; Tang, X.; Chu, L.; Song, Y. Characteristics of cell growth and lipid accumulation of high and low lipid-producing strains of *Mucor circinelloides* grown on different glucose-oil mixed media. *Pro. Biochem.* **2018**, *72*, 31–40. [CrossRef]
43. Tauk-Tornisielo, S.M.; Arasato, L.S.; de-Almeida, A.F.; Govone, J.S.; Malagutti, E.N. Lipid formation and γ-linolenic acid production by *Mucor circinelloides* and *Rhizopus* sp., grown on vegetable oil. *Braz. J. Microbiol.* **2009**, *40*, 342–345. [CrossRef] [PubMed]
44. Du Preez, J.C.; Immelman, M.; Kock, J.L.F.; Kilian, S.G. Production of γ-linolenic acid by *Mucor circinelloides* and *Mucor rouxii* with acetic acid as carbon substrate. *Biotechnol. Lett.* **1995**, *17*, 933–938. [CrossRef]

© 2019 by the authors. Licensee MDPI, Basel, Switzerland. This article is an open access article distributed under the terms and conditions of the Creative Commons Attribution (CC BY) license (http://creativecommons.org/licenses/by/4.0/).

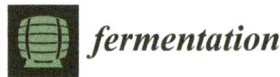

Review

Nutritional and Microbiological Quality of Tiger Nut Tubers (*Cyperus esculentus*), Derived Plant-Based and Lactic Fermented Beverages

Elena Roselló-Soto [1], Cyrielle Garcia [2], Amandine Fessard [2], Francisco J. Barba [1], Paulo E. S. Munekata [3], Jose M. Lorenzo [3] and Fabienne Remize [2,*]

[1] Nutrition and Food Science Area, Preventive Medicine and Public Health, Food Science, Toxicology and Forensic Medicine Department, Universitat de València, Avda. Vicent Andrés Estellés, s/n 46100 Burjassot, València, Spain; eroso2@alumni.uv.es (E.R.-S); francisco.barba@uv.es (F.J.B.)

[2] QualiSud, Université de La Réunion, CIRAD, Université Montpellier, Montpellier SupAgro, Université d'Avignon, 2 rue J. Wetzell, F-97490 Sainte Clotilde, France; cyrielle.garcia@univ-reunion.fr (C.G.); amandine.fessard@hotmail.fr (A.F.)

[3] Centro Tecnológico de la Carne de Galicia, rúa Galicia n 4, Parque Tecnológico de Galicia, 32900 San Cibrao das Viñas, Ourense, Spain; pmunekata@gmail.com (P.E.S.M.); jmlorenzo@ceteca.net (J.M.L.)

* Correspondence: fabienne.remize@univ-reunion.fr; Tel.: +262-692-200-785

Received: 12 November 2018; Accepted: 19 December 2018; Published: 20 December 2018

Abstract: Tiger nut (*Cyperus esculentus*) is a tuber that can be consumed raw or processed into beverages. Its nutritional composition shows a high content of lipid and dietary fiber, close to those of nuts, and a high content of starch, like in other tubers. Tiger nuts also contain high levels of phosphorus, calcium, and phenolic compounds, which contribute to their antioxidant activity. From those characteristics, tiger nuts and derived beverages are particularly relevant to limit food insecurity in regions where the plant can grow. In Europe and United States, the tiger nut derived beverages are of high interest as alternatives to milk and for gluten-free diets. Fermentation or addition of probiotic cultures to tiger nut beverages has proven the ability of lactic acid bacteria to acidify the beverages. Preliminary sensory assays concluded that acceptable products are obtained. In the absence of pasteurization, the safety of tiger nut-based beverages is not warranted. In spite of fermentation, some foodborne pathogens or mycotoxigenic fungi have been observed in fermented beverages. Further studies are required to select a tailored bacterial cocktail which would effectively dominate endogenous flora, preserve bioactive compounds and result in a well-accepted beverage.

Keywords: tiger nuts; horchata; lactic fermentation; beverage; quality; product development

1. Introduction

Increased consumption of fruits and vegetables is recognized to protect against non-communicable diseases [1,2]. Health benefits of fruit and vegetable intake have been historically related to their high content in vitamins, minerals, and phytochemicals. They are also recommended as a source of dietary fibers. For this purpose, starchy roots and tubers have a considerable role for carbohydrate and dietary fiber intake [3]. This role is of great importance for gluten-free diets, which are characterized by insufficient dietary fiber uptake [4–6]. In addition, comparatively to dairy products, plant-based materials do not contain lactose or dairy allergens and exhibit low cholesterol content. Moreover, they benefit from a vegan-friendly status. Among plant-based alternatives to milk, the most popular are soya, almond- and rice-based beverages, but other substitutes, either directly obtained from traditional edible plant extraction, either fermented, are gaining interest as the market is rapidly expanding [6–8].

Lactic fermentation is a traditional and sustainable way to increase the shelf-life of food products as well as to change texture, flavor, and taste [9,10]. In addition, depending on the bacterial strains, a probiotic effect, defined as a health benefit on the host, conferred by living microorganisms administered in adequate amounts, can be expected [11].

Historically, lactic fermentation has been applied to a variety of raw materials, including milk, meat, fish, cereals, vegetables, and fruits [9,12–14]. Lactic fermentation of cereals, including maize, millet, barley, oats, rye, wheat, rice or sorghum, into beverages is ancestral and commonly used in Africa [7,15]. Lactic fermented beverages obtained from teas or vegetables or fruits, with high functional value, were also described [16,17]. The development of new lactic-fermented products is explored worldwide and is recognized as the most suitable way for increasing the daily consumption of fresh-like vegetables and fruits [7,10,16].

Tiger nut (*Cyperus esculentus*) is a tuber, mainly harvested in Spain, West Africa countries like Nigeria, Senegal, or Ghana, and also in South America, as in Chile [18,19]. From an economic point of view, tiger nut is described as an underutilized African crop with high potential for development [20]. Because of its ecological plasticity and its invasive capacity, this plant is considered as a weed or a crop depending on the context [18]. In West Africa, the tubers are often part of the diet as they are cheap, available all the year around, and with nutritional benefits [20]. Recent market changes show how innovative tiger nut based beverages are arising around Europe and this tuber is becoming popular in the US [21].

Nutritional composition of tiger nut tubers shows some unique features, between other tubers and nuts [19]. Starch content of tiger nut is closely related to that of cassava, whereas lipid and even more fiber contents resemble those found for almonds or pistachios. Its composition and associated health benefits offer to this tuber a huge potential for product development. Nowadays, tubers are consumed raw, roasted or after transformation into beverage or flour. The beverage is obtained after several washing steps to eliminate dusts and poor-quality tubers, soaking overnight the dry tubers in water, disinfection with chlorinated water, blending with water, pressing, and filtering (Figure 1).

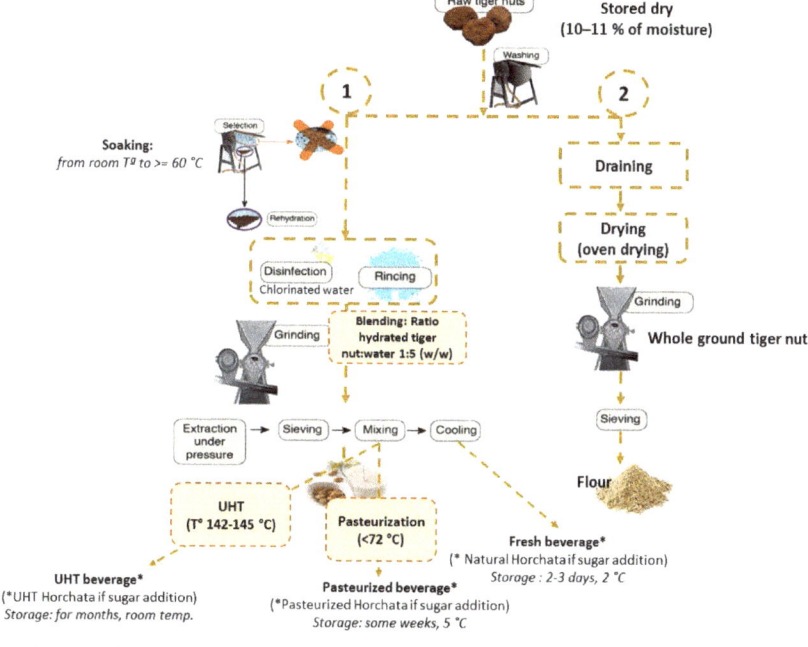

Figure 1. Flowchart showing industrial processing of tiger nuts (1) beverages and (2) flours.

The beverages obtained from this process are called improperly tiger nut milk [22,23] or juice [24]. In Spain, added with a minimum of 10% sugar, this is the very popular drink called "Horchata". Processing this product is regulated: a minimum of 12 Brix, 1.9% of starch, 2% of fats, total sugars expressed as sucrose of 10%, and a pH above 6.3 [25]. Horchata can be produced fresh, pasteurized, sterilized, concentrated or even in powder. When heat treatments are applied, an amylolytic step is required before applying a temperature above 75 °C to avoid starch gelatinization. Whole ground tiger nut and flour are also commercialized. Both the fermentation of tiger nut derived beverage or the addition of probiotic cultures have been evaluated in several studies, resulting in tiger nut yogurts [23,26–31]. Moreover, the "Horchata" production process results in several by-products, such as the drained-water, which is suitable for other applications [32].

This review examines the latest description of nutritional composition, together with microbiological quality, of tiger nuts and derived beverages. We provide a review of the impact of lactic fermentation on the quality of tiger nut beverages. From those data, we focus on the relevance of the consumption of fermented beverages and their potential for new product development.

2. Nutritional Characteristics and Bioactive Compounds of Tiger Nut

The energy value of tiger nut tuber ranges within 400–413.8 kcal/100 g [19,33]. The main components of tiger nut are carbohydrates, which represent 43.3 g/100g. Starch content, 29.9% in wet matter, is similar to that of cassava and about twice that of potato [19]. Dietary fiber content, of 8.81 g/100g, is much higher than in other tubers, which contain 0.66–2.55 g/100g, and in similar ranges than nuts. It is constituted of insoluble dietary fiber at 99.8%. Sucrose content, 13.03 g/100g, is also much higher than in other tubers, ranging from 0.31 to 4.77 g/100g.

Tiger nut contains 22% to 45% of fat in dry matter, depending on the origin of the tubers [34]. In wet matter, due to a higher moisture content of ca. 26%, lipid content is lower than in tree nuts.

The examination of the fat structure in seed oils obtained from tiger nut showed that neutral lipids, dominated by triacylglycerols constitute the bulk of lipids and represent 65.9% of total lipids, while glycolipids and phospholipids represent 5.6–6.9% and 1.4–3.1%, respectively. The structural feature is consistent with most vegetable oils, with monounsaturated acids predominantly found in greater amounts at the sn-2 position, and a lower prevalence of saturated fatty acids, located in the sn-1 and sn-3 positions [35,36]. The main fatty acids are oleic 56% to 85%, palmitic 10% to 20%, linoleic 8% to 12% and stearic 0.3% to 5.3% acids [19,34,37,38], while the minor acids were linolenic and palmitoleic [35]. Tiger nuts composition in monounsaturated fatty acids is in agreement to that found for olive oil, being the fatty acid profile used as a possible geographical authenticity marker. Tiger nut naturally contains a number of sterol components that are of a different composition than the components found in olive oil. β-sitosterol was found as the main compound ($\approx$49–60 mg/100g), followed by stigmasterol, campesterol, α and β-tocopherols [39].

Protein content in tiger nut (5.04–6.67% wet matter) is higher than that found in other tubers, but lower than in nuts. For instance, the protein content of tubers ranges from 0.66% in sweet potato to 2.55% in yam, whereas pine nuts and peanuts contain 13.7% and 25.8% of proteins, respectively [19]. The predominant protein fraction (82–91%) corresponds to the water-soluble fraction of albumin and non-protein nitrogen. The analysis of these fractions by electrophoresis presented a high diversity in polypeptide molecular weights, highlighted at 20, 25, 37, 55, 75 and $\sim$106 kDa. The other solubilized fractions of globulins (1.11–3.96%), prolamins (0.91–3.45%) and glutelins (0.63–1.98%) presented a pattern with fewer different molecular weight polypeptides [40]. The amino acid profile shows, in decreasing order, aspartic acid, glutamic acid, leucine, alanine and arginine [37]. In addition to protein anabolism, L-Arginine is of particular interest as it is the main precursor of nitric oxide (NO), a non-adrenergic and non-cholinergic neurotransmitter involved in numerous physiological and signaling processes, with a strong vasodilator action. For instance, a dried defatted tiger nut tuber dietary supplementation of rats fed with L-NAME nitric oxide synthase inhibitor (Nω-nitro-L-arginine methyl ester hydrochloride) presented an effect on NO metabolism, preventing the reduction in the production of nitric oxide synthesis markers in serum and penile tissue. It also prevented the increased activity of enzymes like acetylcholinesterase, arginase, and adenosine deaminase, leading to the inhibition of NO production whether on serum, on brain or on penile tissue [41].

Tiger nut tubers exhibit high calcium, and phosphorus mineral contents [33,34,37]. On the other hand, magnesium, manganese, iron, zinc and copper are also present, but at lower levels.

Apart from those main characteristics, phenolic and anti-nutrient compounds were analyzed [38,42,43] (Table 1). Phytates represented ≈21.4 mg/100g in raw tubers, oxalates ≈13.1 mg/100g, alkaloids ≈2.6 mg/100g and tannins ≈2.4 mg/100g. The content of all these families of compounds was decreased after soaking, with a more marked effect when soaking was performed at 60 °C/7h compared to room temperature 12h [42]. The highest decrease was observed for tannins (61%), followed by oxalates with (58%) and polyphenols (48%). The main discrepancies were observed with the data published by Chukwuma et al. (2010) [43], but for tannins, phytates and polyphenols, the contents were 100-fold below those observed in other tubers or in chickpeas [44–46]. The composition analysis shows that *trans*-ferulic acid, vanillic acid, vanillin and *trans*-cinnamic acid are the main phenolic compounds in tiger nut oils [38]. Moreover, the antioxidant activity of tiger nut polyphenols was investigated in comparison with flavonoids from a chemoprotective perspective. A dietary supplementation with 25% of whole tiger nut showed moderate renal and hepatoprotective properties against acrylamide-induced toxicity in rats [47].

Table 1. Phenolic profile of tiger nut.

Compound	Concentration	Ref.
Apigenin	7.91–50.58 mg GAE/100 g	[48]
Caffeic acid	1.07–15.25 mg GAE/100 g	[48]
	3.90–102.19 µg RE/kg	[49]
(Epi)Catechin	8.83×10^{-4} – 6.58 mg GAE/100 g	[48]
Cinnamic acid	0–40.66 µg RE/kg	[49]
Coumaric acid	0–6801.0 µg/g	[50]
	4.20×10^{-4} – 17.25 mg GAE/100 g	[48]
	0–126.76 µg RE/kg	[49]
Ferulic acid	3.5–2,284 µg/g	[50]
	33.79–58.38 mg GAE/100 g	[48]
	0–22.33 µg RE/kg	[49]
Diferulic acid	0.0–829.0 µg/g	[50]
Ferulic acid-4-O-glucoside	0–46.95 µg RE/kg	[49]
Gallic acid	3.95×10^{-3} – 1.74 mg GAE/100 g	[48]
Homovanillyl alcohol	0–4.54 µg RE/kg	[49]
p-Hydroxybenzaldehyde	0–16.47 mg GAE/100 g	[48]
	4.0–337.0 µg/g	[50]
p-Hydroxybenzoic acid	0–8.3 µg/g	[50]
	2.18–29.12 mg GAE/100 g	[48]
	2.52–67.70 µg RE/kg	[49]
Isohydroxymatairesinol	0–1331.45	[49]
Kaempferol	3.62–24.44 mg GAE/100 g	[48]
Luteolin	7.29–72.17 mg GAE/100 g	[48]
24-Methylcholestanol ferulate	0–45.40 µg RE/kg	[49]
Naringenin	2.38×10^{-3} – 16.16 mg GAE/100 g	[48]
Peonidin	0–7.81 µg RE/kg	[49]
Protocatechuic acid	0.61–0.79 mg GAE/100 g	[48]
Quercetin	3.76×10^{-3}-60.63 mg GAE/100 g	[48]
trans-Resveratrol-3-O-glucoside	0–25.68 µg RE/kg	[49]
Scopoletin	0–310.80 µg RE/kg	[49]
Sesamin	0–28.67 µg RE/kg	[49]
Sinapinic acid	8.53×10^{-1} – 20.97 mg GAE/100 g	[48]

Table 1. Cont.

Compound	Concentration	Ref.
Sinensetin	0–16.07 µg RE/kg	[49]
Syringic acid	4.58×10^{-4} – 4.12 mg GAE/100 g	[48]
Vanillic acid	3.0–25.3 µg/g	[50]
	5.88–15.20 mg GAE/100 g	[48]
	0–10.84 µg RE/kg	[49]
Vanillin	15.5–68.7 µg/g	[50]
ethyl Vanillin	0–25.38 µg RE/kg	[49]
4-Vinylphenol	0–1084.48 µg RE/kg	[49]

GAE: Gallic Acid Equivalent; RE: resveratrol Equivalent.

3. Nutritional Characteristics of Tiger Nut-Based Beverages

The main composition of tiger nut-based beverages, i.e., Horchata de Chufa and juices, is presented in Table 2.

Table 2. Proximate major nutritional content in tiger nut tubers and beverages.

Nutrient	Tiger Nut Tuber (g/100g) [a]	Horchata De Chufa (g/100g) [a]	Tiger Nut Beverage (g/100g)	
Total fat	24.49	3.09	1.26–1.59 [b]	1.88–2.27 [c]
SFA (% total fatty acid)	17.5			
MUFA (% total fatty acid)	72.9			
PUFA (% total fatty acid)	9.3			
Ratio n-6/n-3	22			
Proteins	5.04	0.91	2.34–2.51 [b]	0.47–0.54 [c]
Ash	1.7	0.25	0.31–0.39 [b]	0.16–0.18 [c]
Carbohydrates	43.3	nd	1.93–2.34 [b]	2.31–2.74 [c]
Total dietary fiber	8.91	1.03	0.23–0.31 [b]	0.53–0.65 [c]
Sucrose	13.03	>10		
Total energy (kcal/100g)	413.8	>71.45	28.42–33.71 [b]	28.04–33.55 [c]

[a] data from Sanchez-Zapata 2012 [19], Horchata de Chufa was prepared from tiger nut beverage and additives including more than 10% of sucrose; [b] Tiger nut beverage was obtained by soaking Nigerian tiger nut in water (1:3 w/v) for 10 h, then by blending drained nuts with water (1:5 w/v). The resulting homogenous slurry was filtered using a muslin cloth and the resultant filtrate was pasteurized at 67 °C for 30 min [24]; [c] To obtain tiger nut beverage, tiger nut from Ghana were first dried for two months at room temperature. The nuts were hydrated by soaking in a water bath for 24 h at 40 °C then grinded with water (1:4 w/v). Finer particles were obtained by dispersing the sample with ultra-turrax mixer at 13,000 rpm for 20 min and were then transferred into a pneumatic press using one volume of water, to be filtered through a 4 µm-pore-size filter membrane [51]; SFA: saturated fatty acids; MUFA: monounsaturated fatty acids; PUFA: polyunsaturated fatty acids; nd: not determined value.

As can be seen in the table, tiger nut beverage, which differed from that of "Horchata" in the fact that there is no sucrose addition, exhibits energy values ranging from 28.42 to 33.55 kcal/100 mL [19,42]. These values are close to those of skim cow milk (33 kcal/100 mL), and in the early window by comparison with soy-based "milk" alternatives, which range from 33 to 58 kcal/100 mL. The overall plant-based "milk" alternatives present a larger range (12–92 kcal/100 mL).

A protein content between 0.47–2.51% can be expected in tiger nut beverages according to the process of extraction [24,51]. Considering the plant-based "milk" alternatives, the highest overall protein content is found in soy-based beverages, ranging from 2.50 to 3.16% whether rice and almond-based "milk" alternatives exhibit the lowest protein content with 0.28% and 0.31–0.59%, respectively [52]. The tiger nut beverage concentration of essential amino acids is 14.27 g/100 g of proteins, which represents ≈28% of the total amino acid content. It can be observed that leucine is the limiting amino acid [24]. Although the tiger nut beverage amino acid scores are lower than the few existing values, namely for quinoa or soy, which have amino acid scores all above 100%, the essential amino acid composition is of interest and differs from some other plant-based beverage proteins.

Methionine and cysteine show a relative abundance in tiger nut whereas they are the limiting amino acids in pea, almond and soy proteins [52]. The calculation of tiger nut beverage amino acid score values [53] ranged from 29% for leucine to 87% for methionine plus cysteine for infants/pre-school children, and 31% to 102% respectively for adults.

The fat content of tiger nut tuber is far above those of beverages, and as expected from tuber composition, the lipid fraction is mainly composed of oleic, palmitic, and linoleic acids. Interestingly, the fractionation of compounds between beverage and residue fraction is dependent on the compound family, being approximately 4:1 for protein, lipid, salts, and soluble fiber, whereas it is 1:6 for insoluble fiber and 1:1 for carbohydrates [51].

Tiger nut beverage is an emulsion of oil droplets in an aqueous phase and contains starch granules and small solid particles [25]. Starch granules are related to product stability, in particular regarding color and texture. For that matter, a maximal pasteurization temperature is recommended to avoid starch gelatinization [54]. Milling conditions were shown to modulate colloidal stability of the beverage [51]. The stability of the system is ensured by proteins, located at the interphase oil-water. The addition of emulsifiers could be required for long-term storage of the beverage. For instance, the analysis of 87 samples, either fresh artisanal-made, or UHT-treated in industry, revealed that emulsifiers like citric acid esters of mono- or diglycerides, and monoacyl glycerol, are present into industrial tiger nut beverages. On the opposite, phosphatidic acid is present only in fresh beverage, and the fresh beverage content of biotin and of L-arginine is respectively 4-fold and 10-fold higher than in UHT beverage [55].

4. Products Obtained by Lactic Fermentation or Lactic Acid Bacteria Addition

Until now, lactic fermentation of tiger nut beverages has been poorly investigated compared to its multiple interesting applications (e.g., from a nutritional point of view and for new product development). Fermentation of non-dairy beverages has been mainly focused on vegetable juices [56], fruits juices [17,57–60], cereal-based beverages [7,59], but also walnut and cashew nut beverages [61,62]. Although the demand for plant-based milk substitutes is increasing, the unwillingness of the mainstream consumer to try unfamiliar foods that are perceived as unappealing may be a limiting factor. Some undesired flavors could efficiently be reduced by fermentation and the flavor could be more appreciated in presence of lactic acid [8]. Lactic acid bacteria not only modify sensory characteristics of the beverages, but also can produce additional micronutrients [63,64] or increase antioxidant properties [17], produce texturing compounds like exopolysaccharides [65,66], or limit undesirable microorganism development [67–69].

Besides lactic fermentation of foods and beverages, the addition of lactic acid bacteria cultures *per se* can bring numerous advantages by the production of compounds, like exopolysaccharides, which modify the texture [6]. The use of probiotic lactic acid bacteria to develop new functional beverages from fruits or vegetables is challenging, because the growth or survival of bacteria in such media has to be carefully examined [70–75]. But the interest is even more significant for food matrices that contain a high content of dietary fiber, and can serve as a prebiotic [71,75]. For developing countries, the selection of probiotic bacteria can be an issue to limit food insecurity [76].

The first study reporting tiger nut beverage fermentation compared the obtained product with cow milk yogurt [29]. Classical yogurt starters were used, i.e., *Lactobacillus bulgaricus* and *Streptococcus thermophilus*, to ferment tiger nut beverage. As expected, the fermentation resulted into an acidified product, at a pH of 3.9, which was overall less appreciated by a small untrained panel than the classical yogurt. Ukwuru et al. (2008) could not detect any difference of general acceptability between fermented tiger nut beverage and cow milk [30], but the lower acceptability of yogurt-processed tiger nut beverage compared to classical cow milk yogurt was confirmed by Sanful et al. (2009) with a broader sensory panel [31]. At this stage, the production of a fermented product from a 1:1 mix of tiger nut and cow milks seems to be the best compromise for sensory attributes, but this product loses the advantages of a plant-based yogurt.

Tiger nut beverage fermentation performed with a *Lactobacillus plantarum* isolated from spontaneous fermentation demonstrated the ability of this strain to grow and to acidify the beverage [27]. Interestingly, an attempt to ferment tiger nut beverage with isolates from *Ogi*, a traditional fermented cereal porridge from Nigeria, resulted in a pH decrease up to 4.04–4.36 depending on isolated combinations [23]. In that study, four species (*Lb. plantarum*, *Lactobacillus acidophilus*, *St. thermophilus* and *Lactobacillus brevis*) were used, and three combinations of three isolates among those bacteria were used, resulting into comparable growth and acidification levels.

None of the previous studies reported a phase separation over fermentation. However, this could be expected from its composition, as the stability of this complex system depends on oil-water droplets, the protein emulsifying effect, and small solid particles. Acidification would modify protein surface properties. Moreover, in fermented non-dairy beverages, the role of exopolysaccharides, produced by bacteria, on texture and sensory quality has been demonstrated for a long time [77,78]. The use of exopolysaccharides producing lactic acid bacteria demonstrated their positive impact on the texture of fermented soy beverages [79] and on pureed carrots [80]. A similar approach would be of great interest for tiger nut beverages. Moreover, exopolysaccharides exert some beneficial health effects [81].

The role of proteins in beverage stability and the interest in protein fortification of food encouraged the formulation of fermented beverages from tiger nuts supplemented with soybean, sorghum, whey proteins, and caseinate [28,82]. Xanthan gum was also used for its thickening and stabilization effects [28]. A beverage containing sorghum, soybean, and tiger nut flours in ratio 5:3:2 and fermented with *Lb. plantarum* exhibited a decrease of counts of yeasts and molds and of enterobacteria below the detection limit over 24h of fermentation. This beverage contained 26.6% of proteins and 26.2% of carbohydrates on a wet base, and was positively evaluated by a sensory panel [82]. Dairy protein addition modified gel properties, leading to semi-solid, yogurt-like gels [28]. Gel stiffness and viscosity were higher and whey drainage was lower when sodium caseinate was used instead of whey proteins, hence opening a way for texture modulation by varying the protein type and content.

Compared to other lactic fermented beverages with a plant-origin, there are some features observed in the original nutritional composition of tiger nut beverages. The natural balance in good quality nutrients, likewise, unsaturated fat, minerals, and antioxidant, make tiger nut fermented beverages a potential candidate for diet complementation. The abundance of unsaturated fatty acids together with antioxidant compounds is an effective choice for lowering the dietary intake of saturated fatty acids and to limit oxidative stress. Oleic acid especially is suggested to reverse induced hyperlipidemia and to have a strong hepatoprotective effect on rats receiving a high fat/high cholesterol diet [83,84]. Depending on the process flow and the final protein content of tiger nut beverages, the determination of protein bioavailability is definitely required to evaluate the effect of lactic fermentation on these nutrients. Tiger nut beverage calcium content of 40 mg/100g is higher than other unfortified milk alternatives having drastically lower contents of calcium, ranging from 0 to 12 mg/100 g [52]. The calcium bioavailability in plant-based beverages is however uncertainly comparable with the 120 mg/100 g cow milk calcium content, because its natural association with caseins facilitates absorption and limits sedimentation. Whether fermentation improves this parameter, it is also worth further investigation.

Tiger nut composition showed the presence of numerous phenolic compounds. However, the impact of lactic fermentation on these compounds in tiger nut beverages has never been investigated.

5. Safety and Microbiological Quality

In a study evaluating the parasite presence of raw tubers collected from street vendors and market places in Ghana, several parasites were found; *Cryptosporidium parvum* being the most common [85]. Enterobacteria and *Staphylococcus* sp. were also detected. Moreover, several species of mycotoxin-producing molds, *Aspergillus niger*, *Aspergillus fumigatus*, *Aspergillus flavus* and *Penicillium italicum*, were found in raw tiger nut tubers [27]. Mycotoxins were detected in both raw tiger nuts and beverages [86,87]. Aflatoxins B_1 and G_2, beauvericin and ochratoxin A were the predominant mycotoxins detected in tubers, with respectively 14, 10, 11 and 8 samples upon 83 that exhibited toxin contents over the limits of quantification.

The pH of tiger nut beverage is in the range 6.3–6.8 [19], which is not limiting the growth of food-borne pathogens. On tiger nut beverage samples, two microbiological profiles were observed depending on the process applied, either industrial or home-made [88]. On industrial products, which were heat-treated, no foodborne pathogen could be detected, and total viable bacteria counts were below the detection limit. On the opposite, the home-made products exhibited total viable counts in the range of 3.6–6.5 log CFU/mL, and on certain samples, enterobacteria, *Bacillus* sp., *Escherichia coli* and yeast and molds were found. In another study [30], an increase of bacterial counts from 1.3 log CFU/mL to 3.5 log CFU/mL and 8.5 log CFU/mL, when stored at 4 °C or at 32 °C respectively, was observed after 6 days of storage. The samples stored at 32 °C showed spoilage signs after 6 days. The refrigerated sample remained drinkable over 14 days and the bacterial counts reached then 4.4 log CFU/mL.

In tiger nut beverage, ochratoxin A was detected in 32 samples from 238, but below quantification limit. Aflatoxins B1, B2 and G2 were detected in 12, 2 and 1 samples, respectively from 238, and below the maximal limits fixed by EU.

Fermentation generally results in an increase of safety thanks to acidification and to the production of bacteriostatic compounds such as organic acids, hydrogen peroxide or bacteriocins [9,89]. Lactic acid bacteria also can impair the growth of mycotoxin-producing fungi, inhibit the biosynthesis of mycotoxins or degrade the compounds [89–91]. Only preliminary studies have investigated safety or the microbiological quality of the fermented tiger nut beverages. Agbaje et al. (2015) [27] isolated and identified potential foodborne pathogens, such as *Staphylococcus aureus*, and mycotoxinogen fungi. Traditional fermented beverages hold their own microbial ecosystem, among those lactic acid bacteria are diverse and often associated with yeasts [7,59,92]. To date, contrarily to other fermented vegetables [93–96], there is no data on tiger nut beverage microbiota.

6. Conclusions and Future Research for Functional Beverages and Foods

The interest in the lactic fermentation of plant-based beverages emerged from the search of "substitutes" to milk, due to the allergenicity or vegan-based considerations. In developing countries, the objective to fulfill nutritional requirements of people affected by food insecurity is another leading reason for this type of research. Most of these studies highlighted the value of developing featured tastes and flavors, together with an increased shelf-life of perishable products. In line with that objective, the development of fermented products from tiger nut beverages is particularly relevant.

The requirement of starters isolated from a similar origin is pointed out as a key-factor for successful fermentation [97–99]. When developing new fermented beverages from plant-origin, the choice for fermentative bacteria selected from fermented plants should be recommended. Moreover, the selection of tailored microbial starters contributes to the safety of the fermented foods and beverages by two aspects: i) the safety of the starter itself, ensured by its GRAS status and not producing toxic compounds, and ii) its ability to decrease hazards in a given food or beverage [100]. Consequently, extensive research on lactic acid bacterial starters adapted to tiger nut beverage fermentation is still required.

Funding: This work was supported by Federation BioST of the University of La Reunion and European Union project RE0017203 and the project GV/2018//040 "Implementación y optimización de procesos innovadores para la valorización de los subproductos obtenidos a partir del proceso de elaboración de la horchata" for emerging research groups from the Generalitat Valenciana. Paulo E. Munekata acknowledges the postdoctoral fellowship support from the Ministry of Economy and Competitiveness (MINECO, Spain) "Juan de la Cierva" program (FJCI-2016-29486).

Conflicts of Interest: The authors declare no conflict of interest. The funding sponsors had no role in the writing of the manuscript, and in the decision to publish.

References

1. Slavin, J.L.; Lloyd, B. Health benefits of fruits and vegetables. *Adv. Nutr.* **2012**, *3*, 506–516. [CrossRef] [PubMed]
2. Nishida, C.; Uauy, R.; Kumanyika, S.; Shetty, P. The Joint WHO/FAO Expert Consultation on diet, nutrition and the prevention of chronic diseases: Process, product and policy implications. *Public Health Nutr.* **2004**, *7*, 245–250. [CrossRef] [PubMed]
3. Chandrasekara, A.; Josheph Kumar, T. Roots and tuber crops as functional foods: A review on phytochemical constituents and their potential health benefits. *Int. J. Food Sci.* **2016**, *2016*, 1–15. [CrossRef] [PubMed]
4. Wild, D.; Robins, G.G.; Burley, V.J.; Howdle, P.D. Evidence of high sugar intake, and low fibre and mineral intake, in the gluten-free diet. *Aliment. Pharmacol. Ther.* **2010**, *32*, 573–581. [CrossRef]
5. Vici, G.; Belli, L.; Biondi, M.; Polzonetti, V. Gluten free diet and nutrient deficiencies: A review. *Clin. Nutr.* **2016**, *35*, 1236–1241. [CrossRef]
6. Jeske, S.; Arendt, E.K. Past, present and future: The strength of plant-based dairy substitutes based on gluten-free raw materials. *Food Res. Int.* **2018**, *110*, 42–51. [CrossRef]
7. Marsh, A.J.; Hill, C.; Ross, R.P.; Cotter, P.D. Fermented beverages with health-promoting potential: Past and future perspectives. *Trends Food Sci. Technol.* **2014**, *38*, 113–124. [CrossRef]
8. Mäkinen, O.E.; Wanhalinna, V.; Zannini, E.; Arendt, E.K. Foods for special dietary needs: Non-dairy plant-based milk substitutes and fermented dairy-type products. *Crit. Rev. Food Sci. Nutr.* **2016**, *56*, 339–349. [CrossRef] [PubMed]
9. Caplice, E.; Fitzgerald, G.F. Food fermentations: Role of microorganisms in food production and preservation. *Int. J. Food Microbiol.* **1999**, *50*, 131–149. [CrossRef]
10. Hugenholtz, J. Traditional biotechnology for new foods and beverages. *Curr. Opin. Biotechnol.* **2013**, *24*, 155–159. [CrossRef]
11. Hill, C.; Guarner, F.; Reid, G.; Gibson, G.R.; Merenstein, D.J.; Pot, B.; Morelli, L.; Canani, R.B.; Flint, H.J.; Salminen, S.; et al. The International Scientific Association for Probiotics and Prebiotics consensus statement on the scope and appropriate use of the term probiotic. *Nat. Rev. Gastroenterol. Hepatol.* **2014**, *11*, 506–514. [CrossRef] [PubMed]
12. Oyewole, O.B. Lactic fermented foods in Africa and their benefits. *Food Control* **1997**, *8*, 289–297. [CrossRef]
13. Lee, C.-H. Lactic acid fermented foods and their benefits in Asia. *Food Control* **1997**, *8*, 259–269. [CrossRef]
14. Tamang, J.P.; Watanabe, K.; Holzapfel, W.H. Review: Diversity of microorganisms in global fermented foods and beverages. *Front. Microbiol.* **2016**, *7*, 377. [CrossRef] [PubMed]
15. Blandino, A.; Al-Aseeri, M.E.; Pandiella, S.S.; Cantero, D.; Webb, C. Cereal-based fermented foods and beverages. *Food Res. Int.* **2003**, *36*, 527–543. [CrossRef]
16. Di Cagno, R.; Coda, R.; De Angelis, M.; Gobbetti, M. Exploitation of vegetables and fruits through lactic acid fermentation. *Food Microbiol.* **2013**, *33*, 1–10. [CrossRef] [PubMed]
17. Fessard, A.; Kapoor, A.; Patche, J.; Assemat, S.; Hoarau, M.; Bourdon, E.; Bahorun, T.; Remize, F. Lactic fermentation as an efficient tool to enhance the antioxidant activity of tropical fruit juices and teas. *Microorganisms* **2017**, *5*, 23. [CrossRef]
18. De Castro, O.; Gargiulo, R.; Del Guacchio, E.; Caputo, P.; De Luca, P. A molecular survey concerning the origin of *Cyperus esculentus* (Cyperaceae, Poales): Two sides of the same coin (weed vs. crop). *Ann. Bot.* **2015**, *115*, 733–745. [CrossRef]
19. Sánchez-Zapata, E.; Fernández-López, J.; Angel Pérez-Alvarez, J. Tiger nut (*Cyperus esculentus*) commercialization: Health aspects, composition, properties, and food applications. *Compr. Rev. Food Sci. Food Saf.* **2012**, *11*, 366–377. [CrossRef]
20. Bamishaiye, E.; Bamishaiye, O. Tiger nut: As a plant, its derivatives and benefits. *Afr. J. Food Agric. Nutr. Dev.* **2011**, *11*, 5157–5170. [CrossRef]
21. Van Wyk, B.-E. The potential of South African plants in the development of new food and beverage products. *S. Afr. J. Bot.* **2011**, *77*, 857–868. [CrossRef]
22. Belewu, M.A.; Belewu, K. Comparative physicochemical evaluation of tigernut, soybean and coconut milk sources. *Int. J. Agric. Biol.* **2007**, *9*, 785–787.
23. Maduka, N.; Ire, F.; Njoku, H. Fermentation of tigernut by lactic acid bacteria and tigernut-milk drink fermentation by lactic acid bacteria as a potential probiotic product. *Asian J. Sci. Technol.* **2017**, *8*, 5167–5172.

24. Oa, O. Determination of amino acids and physico-chemical properties of juice samples produced from five varieties of tigernut (*Cyperus esculentus*). *Chem. Res. J.* **2016**, *1*, 1–6.
25. Codina, I.; Trujillo, A.J.; Ferragut, V. Horchata. In *Traditional Foods*; Springer: Boston, MA, USA, 2016; pp. 345–356.
26. Sánchez-Zapata, E.; Fernández-López, J.; Pérez-Alvarez, J.A.; Soares, J.; Sousa, S.; Gomes, A.M.P.; Pintado, M.M.E. In vitro evaluation of "horchata" co-products as carbon source for probiotic bacteria growth. *Food Bioprod. Process.* **2013**, *91*, 279–286. [CrossRef]
27. Agbaje, R.B.; Oyetayo, O.V.; Ojokoh, A.O. Assessment of the microbial and physico-chemical composition of tigernut subjected to different fermentation methods. *Pak. J. Nutr.* **2015**, *14*, 742–748. [CrossRef]
28. Kizzie-Hayford, N.; Jaros, D.; Zahn, S.; Rohm, H. Effects of protein enrichment on the microbiological, physicochemical and sensory properties of fermented tiger nut milk. *LWT Food Sci. Technol.* **2016**, *74*, 319–324. [CrossRef]
29. Akoma, O.; Elekwa, U.O.; Afodunrinbi, A.T.; Onyeukwu, G.C. Yogurt from Coconut and Tigernuts. *J. Food Technol. Afr.* **2000**, *5*, 132–134. [CrossRef]
30. Ukwuru, M. Production and quality assessment of tiger nut (*Cyperus esculentus*) imitation milk during storage. *J. Food Sci. Technol.* **2008**, *45*, 180–182.
31. Sanful, R.E. The use of tiger-nut (*Cyperus esculentus*), cow milk and their composite as substrates for yoghurt production. *Pak. J. Nutr.* **2009**, *8*, 755–758. [CrossRef]
32. Sánchez-Zapata, E.; Fuentes-Zaragoza, E.; Viuda-Martos, M.; Fernández-López, J.; Sendra, E.; Sayas, E.; Pérez-Alvarez, J.A. Reclaim of the by-products from "Horchata" elaboration process. *Food Bioprocess Technol.* **2012**, *5*, 954–963. [CrossRef]
33. USDA Branded Food Products Database. Available online: https://ndb.nal.usda.gov/ndb/ (accessed on 26 November 2018).
34. Roselló-Soto, E.; Poojary, M.M.; Barba, F.J.; Lorenzo, J.M.; Mañes, J.; Moltó, J.C. Tiger nut and its by-products valorization: From extraction of oil and valuable compounds to development of new healthy products. *Innov. Food Sci. Emerg. Technol.* **2018**, *45*, 306–312. [CrossRef]
35. Kim, M.; No, S.; Yoon, S.H. Stereospecific analysis of fatty acid composition of Chufa (*Cyperus esculentus* L.) tuber oil. *J. Am. Oil Chem. Soc.* **2007**, *84*, 1079–1080. [CrossRef]
36. Yeboah, S.O.; Mitei, Y.C.; Ngila, J.C.; Wessjohann, L.; Schmidt, J. Compositional and structural studies of the oils from two edible seeds: Tiger nut, *Cyperus esculentum*, and asiato, *Pachira insignis*, from Ghana. *Food Res. Int.* **2012**, *47*, 259–266. [CrossRef]
37. Arafat, S.; Gaafar, A.; Basuny, A.M.; Nassef, S. Chufa tubers (*Cyperus esculentus* L.) as a new source of food. *World Appl. Sci. J.* **2009**, *7*, 151–156.
38. Ezeh, O.; Niranjan, K.; Gordon, M.H. Effect of enzyme pre-treatments on bioactive compounds in extracted tiger nut oil and sugars in residual meals. *J. Am. Oil Chem. Soc.* **2016**, *93*, 1541–1549. [CrossRef] [PubMed]
39. Lopéz-Cortés, I.; Salazar-García, D.C.; Malheiro, R.; Guardiola, V.; Pereira, J.A. Chemometrics as a tool to discriminate geographical origin of *Cyperus esculentus* L. based on chemical composition. *Ind. Crops Prod.* **2013**, *51*, 19–25. [CrossRef]
40. Codina-Torrella, I.; Guamis, B.; Trujillo, A.J. Characterization and comparison of tiger nuts (*Cyperus esculentus* L.) from different geographical origin: Physico-chemical characteristics and protein fractionation. *Ind. Crops Prod.* **2015**, *65*, 406–414. [CrossRef]
41. Olabiyi, A.A.; Carvalho, F.B.; Bottari, N.B.; Lopes, T.F.; da Costa, P.; Stefanelo, N.; Morsch, V.M.; Akindahunsi, A.A.; Oboh, G.; Schetinger, M.R. Dietary supplementation of tiger nut alters biochemical parameters relevant to erectile function in L-NAME treated rats. *Food Res. Int.* **2018**, *109*, 358–367. [CrossRef]
42. Adekanmi, O.K.; Oluwatooyin, O.F.; Yemisi, A.A. Influence of processing techniques on the nutrients and antinutrients of tigernut (*Cyperus esculentus* L.). *World J. Dairy Food Sci.* **2009**, *4*, 88–93.
43. Ekeanyanwu, R.C.; Njoku, O.; Ononogbu, I.C. The phytochemical composition and some biochemical effects of Nigerian tigernut (*Cyperus esculentus* L.) tuber. *Pak. J. Nutr.* **2010**, *9*, 709–715. [CrossRef]
44. El-Adawy, T.A. Nutritional composition and antinutritional factors of chickpeas (*Cicer arietinum* L.) undergoing different cooking methods and germination. *Plant Foods Hum. Nutr.* **2002**, *57*, 83–97. [CrossRef] [PubMed]
45. Ezeocha, V.; Ojimelukwe, P. The impact of cooking on the proximate composition and anti-nutritional factors of water yam (*Dioscorea alata*). *J. Stored Prod. Postharvest Res.* **2012**, *3*, 172–176. [CrossRef]

46. Omoruyi, F.O.; Dilworth, L.; Asemota, H.N. Anti-nutritional factors, zinc, iron and calcium in some Caribbean tuber crops and the effect of boiling or roasting. *Nutr. Food Sci.* **2007**, *37*, 8–15. [CrossRef]
47. Hamdy, S.M.; Shabaan, A.M.; Abdel Latif, A.K.M.; Abdel-Aziz, A.M.; Amin, A.M. Protective effect of hesperidin and tiger nut against acrylamide toxicity in female rats. *Exp. Toxicol. Pathol.* **2017**, *69*, 580–588. [CrossRef] [PubMed]
48. Oladele, A.K.; Adebowale, J.O.; Bamidele, O.P. Phenolic profile and antioxidant activity of brown and yellow varieties of tigernut (*Cyperus esculentus* L.). *Niger. Food J.* **2017**, *35*, 51–59.
49. Roselló-Soto, E.; Barba, F.J.; Lorenzo, J.M.; Munekata, P.E.S.; Gómez, B.; Moltó, J.C. Phenolic profile of oils obtained from "horchata" by-products assisted by supercritical-CO_2 and its relationship with antioxidant and lipid oxidation parameters: Triple TOF-LC-MS-MS characterization. *Food Chem.* **2019**, *274*, 865–871. [CrossRef] [PubMed]
50. Parker, M.L.; Ng, A.; Smith, A.C.; Waldron, K.W. Esterified phenolics of the cell walls of Chufa (*Cyperus esculentus* L.) tubers and their role in texture. *J. Agric. Food Chem.* **2000**, *48*, 6284–6291. [CrossRef] [PubMed]
51. Kizzie-Hayford, N.; Jaros, D.; Schneider, Y.; Rohm, H. Characteristics of tiger nut milk: Effects of milling. *Int. J. Food Sci. Technol.* **2015**, *50*, 381–388. [CrossRef]
52. Chalupa-Krebzdak, S.; Long, C.J.; Bohrer, B.M. Nutrient density and nutritional value of milk and plant-based milk alternatives. *Int. Dairy J.* **2018**, *87*, 84–92. [CrossRef]
53. FAO/WHO. FAO expert consultation. Dietary protein quality evaluation in human nutrition. In *FAO Food and Nutrition Paper*; FAO/WHO: Auckland, New Zealand, 2013; Vol. 92, p. 19. ISBN 9789251074176.
54. Roselló-Soto, E.; Poojary, M.M.; Barba, F.J.; Koubaa, M.; Lorenzo, J.M.; Mañes, J.; Moltó, J.C. Thermal and non-thermal preservation techniques of tiger nuts' beverage "horchata de chufa". Implications for food safety, nutritional and quality properties. *Food Res. Int.* **2018**, *105*, 945–951. [CrossRef] [PubMed]
55. Rubert, J.; Monforte, A.; Hurkova, K.; Pérez-Martínez, G.; Blesa, J.; Navarro, J.L.; Stranka, M.; Soriano, J.M.; Hajslova, J. Untargeted metabolomics of fresh and heat treatment Tiger nut (*Cyperus esculentus* L.) milks reveals further insight into food quality and nutrition. *J. Chromatogr. A* **2017**, *1514*, 80–87. [CrossRef] [PubMed]
56. Corona, O.; Randazzo, W.; Miceli, A.; Guarcello, R.; Francesca, N.; Erten, H.; Moschetti, G.; Settanni, L. Characterization of kefir-like beverages produced from vegetable juices. *LWT Food Sci. Technol.* **2016**, *66*, 572–581. [CrossRef]
57. Septembre-Malaterre, A.; Remize, F.; Poucheret, P. Fruits and vegetables, as a source of nutritional compounds and phytochemicals: Changes in bioactive compounds during lactic fermentation. *Food Res. Int.* **2017**. [CrossRef] [PubMed]
58. Randazzo, W.; Corona, O.; Guarcello, R.; Francesca, N.; Germanà, M.A.; Erten, H.; Moschetti, G.; Settanni, L. Development of new non-dairy beverages from Mediterranean fruit juices fermented with water kefir microorganisms. *Food Microbiol.* **2016**, *54*, 40–51. [CrossRef]
59. Altay, F.; Karbancıoglu-Güler, F.; Daskaya-Dikmen, C. A review on traditional Turkish fermented non-alcoholic beverages: Microbiota, fermentation process and quality characteristics. *Int. J. Food Microbiol.* **2013**, *167*, 44–56. [CrossRef] [PubMed]
60. Filannino, P.; Azzi, L.; Cavoski, I.; Vincentini, O.; Rizzello, C.G.; Gobbetti, M.; Di Cagno, R. Exploitation of the health-promoting and sensory properties of organic pomegranate (*Punica granatum* L.) juice through lactic acid fermentation. *Int. J. Food Microbiol.* **2013**, *163*, 184–192. [CrossRef]
61. Cui, X.-H.; Chen, S.-J.; Wang, Y.; Han, J.-R. Fermentation conditions of walnut milk beverage inoculated with kefir grains. *LWT Food Sci. Technol.* **2013**, *50*, 349–352. [CrossRef]
62. Tabanelli, G.; Pasini, F.; Riciputi, Y.; Vannini, L.; Gozzi, G.; Balestra, F.; Caboni, M.F.; Gardini, F.; Montanari, C. Fermented nut-based vegan food: Characterization of a home made product and scale-up to an industrial pilot-scale production. *J. Food Sci.* **2018**, *83*, 711–722. [CrossRef]
63. Yépez, A.; Russo, P.; Spano, G.; Khomenko, I.; Biasioli, F.; Capozzi, V.; Aznar, R. In situ riboflavin fortification of different kefir-like cereal-based beverages using selected Andean LAB strains. *Food Microbiol.* **2019**, *77*, 61–68. [CrossRef]
64. Capozzi, V.; Russo, P.; Dueñas, M.T.; López, P.; Spano, G. Lactic acid bacteria producing B-group vitamins: A great potential for functional cereals products. *Appl. Microbiol. Biotechnol.* **2012**, *96*, 1383–1394. [CrossRef]

65. Caggianiello, G.; Kleerebezem, M.; Spano, G. Exopolysaccharides produced by lactic acid bacteria: From health-promoting benefits to stress tolerance mechanisms. *Appl. Microbiol. Biotechnol.* **2016**, *100*, 3877–3886. [CrossRef]
66. Galle, S.; Schwab, C.; Arendt, E.; Gänzle, M. Exopolysaccharide-forming *Weissella* strains as starter cultures for sorghum and wheat sourdoughs. *J. Agric. Food Chem.* **2010**, *58*, 5834–5841. [CrossRef] [PubMed]
67. Sathe, S.J.; Nawani, N.N.; Dhakephalkar, P.K.; Kapadnis, B.P. Antifungal lactic acid bacteria with potential to prolong shelf-life of fresh vegetables. *J. Appl. Microbiol.* **2007**, *103*, 2622–2628. [CrossRef] [PubMed]
68. Russo, P.; Arena, M.P.; Fiocco, D.; Capozzi, V.; Drider, D.; Spano, G. *Lactobacillus plantarum* with broad antifungal activity: A promising approach to increase safety and shelf-life of cereal-based products. *Int. J. Food Microbiol.* **2016**. [CrossRef] [PubMed]
69. Trias, R.; Bañeras, L.; Montesinos, E.; Badosa, E. Lactic acid bacteria from fresh fruit and vegetables as biocontrol agents of phytopathogenic bacteria and fungi. *Int. Microbiol.* **2008**, *11*, 231–236. [CrossRef]
70. Min, M.; Bunt, C.R.; Mason, S.L.; Hussain, M.A. Non-dairy probiotic food products: An emerging group of functional foods. *Crit. Rev. Food Sci. Nutr.* **2018**, 1–16. [CrossRef] [PubMed]
71. Salmerón, I. Fermented cereal beverages: From probiotic, prebiotic and synbiotic towards Nanoscience designed healthy drinks. *Lett. Appl. Microbiol.* **2017**, *65*, 114–124. [CrossRef] [PubMed]
72. Mridula, D.; Sharma, M. Development of non-dairy probiotic drink utilizing sprouted cereals, legume and soymilk. *LWT Food Sci. Technol.* **2015**, *62*, 482–487. [CrossRef]
73. Panghal, A.; Janghu, S.; Virkar, K.; Gat, Y.; Kumar, V.; Chhikara, N. Potential non-dairy probiotic products—A healthy approach. *Food Biosci.* **2018**, *21*, 80–89. [CrossRef]
74. Kandylis, P.; Pissaridi, K.; Bekatorou, A.; Kanellaki, M.; Koutinas, A.A. Dairy and non-dairy probiotic beverages. *Curr. Opin. Food Sci.* **2016**, *7*, 58–63. [CrossRef]
75. Corbo, M.R.; Bevilacqua, A.; Petruzzi, L.; Casanova, F.P.; Sinigaglia, M. Functional beverages: The emerging side of functional foods. *Compr. Rev. Food Sci. Food Saf.* **2014**, *13*, 1192–1206. [CrossRef]
76. Gheziel, C.; Russo, P.; Arena, M.P.; Spano, G.; Ouzari, H.-I.; Kheroua, O.; Saidi, D.; Fiocco, D.; Kaddouri, H.; Capozzi, V. Evaluating the probiotic potential of *Lactobacillus plantarum* strains from Algerian infant feces: Towards the design of probiotic starter cultures tailored for developing countries. *Probiotics Antimicrob. Proteins* **2018**, 1–11. [CrossRef] [PubMed]
77. Viana de Souza, J.; Silva Dias, F. Protective, technological, and functional properties of select autochthonous lactic acid bacteria from goat dairy products. *Curr. Opin. Food Sci.* **2017**, *13*, 1–9. [CrossRef]
78. Ruas-Madiedo, P.; Hugenholtz, J.; Zoon, P. An overview of the functionality of exopolysaccharides produced by lactic acid bacteria. *Int. Dairy J.* **2002**, *12*, 163–171. [CrossRef]
79. Li, C.; Li, W.; Chen, X.; Feng, M.; Rui, X.; Jiang, M.; Dong, M. Microbiological, physicochemical and rheological properties of fermented soymilk produced with exopolysaccharide (EPS) producing lactic acid bacteria strains. *LWT Food Sci. Technol.* **2014**, *57*, 477–485. [CrossRef]
80. Juvonen, R.; Honkapää, K.; Maina, N.H.; Shi, Q.; Viljanen, K.; Maaheimo, H.; Virkki, L.; Tenkanen, M.; Lantto, R. The impact of fermentation with exopolysaccharide producing lactic acid bacteria on rheological, chemical and sensory properties of pureed carrots (*Daucus carota* L.). *Int. J. Food Microbiol.* **2015**, *207*, 109–118. [CrossRef] [PubMed]
81. Patel, A.; Prajapati, J. Food and health applications of exopolysaccharides produced by lactic acid bacteria. *Adv. Dairy Res.* **2013**, *1*. [CrossRef]
82. Abdulkadir, M.; Danjuma, J.B. Microbial profile and nutritional quality during the fermentation of cereal based weaning food fortified with soya bean and tiger nut using starter culture. *World Sci. News* **2015**, *24*, 103–115.
83. Chen, X.; Li, L.; Liu, X.; Luo, R.; Liao, G.; Li, L.; Liu, J.; Cheng, J.; Lu, Y.; Chen, Y. Oleic acid protects saturated fatty acid mediated lipotoxicity in hepatocytes and rat of non-alcoholic steatohepatitis. *Life Sci.* **2018**, *203*, 291–304. [CrossRef]
84. Pimentel Duavy, S.M.; Torres Salazar, G.J.; de Oliveira Leite, A.; Ecker, A.; Vargas Barbosa, N. Effect of dietary supplementation with olive and sunflower oils on lipid profile and liver histology in rats fed high cholesterol diet. *Asian Pac. J. Trop. Med.* **2017**, *10*, 539–543. [CrossRef] [PubMed]
85. Ayeh-Kumi, P.F.; Tetteh-Quarcoo, P.B.; Duedu, K.O.; Obeng, A.S.; Addo-Osafo, K.; Mortu, S.; Asmah, R.H. A survey of pathogens associated with *Cyperus esculentus* L (tiger nuts) tubers sold in a Ghanaian city. *BMC Res. Notes* **2014**, *7*, 343. [CrossRef] [PubMed]

86. Rubert, J.; Soler, C.; Mañes, J. Occurrence of fourteen mycotoxins in tiger-nuts. *Food Control* **2012**, *25*, 374–379. [CrossRef]
87. Rubert, J.; Sebastià, N.; Soriano, J.M.; Soler, C.; Mañes, J. One-year monitoring of aflatoxins and ochratoxin A in tiger-nuts and their beverages. *Food Chem.* **2011**, *127*, 822–826. [CrossRef] [PubMed]
88. Sebastià, N.; El-Shenawy, M.; Mañes, J.; Soriano, J.M. Assessment of microbial quality of commercial and home-made tiger-nut beverages. *Lett. Appl. Microbiol.* **2012**, *54*, 299–305. [CrossRef] [PubMed]
89. Juodeikiene, G.; Bartkiene, E.; Viskelis, P.; Urbonaviciene, D.; Eidukonyte, D.; Bobinas, C. *Fermentation Processes Using Lactic Acid Bacteria Producing Bacteriocins for Preservation and Improving Functional Properties of Food Products*; Petre, M., Ed.; InTech: Rijeka, Croatia, 2012; ISBN 978-953-307-820-5.
90. Dalié, D.K.D.; Deschamps, A.M.; Richard-Forget, F. Lactic acid bacteria—Potential for control of mould growth and mycotoxins: A review. *Food Control* **2010**, *21*, 370–380. [CrossRef]
91. Chiocchetti, G.M.; Jadán-Piedra, C.; Monedero, V.; Zúñiga, M.; Vélez, D.; Devesa, V. Use of lactic acid bacteria and yeasts to reduce exposure to chemical food contaminants and toxicity. *Crit. Rev. Food Sci. Nutr.* **2018**, 1–12. [CrossRef]
92. Sõukand, R.; Pieroni, A.; Biró, M.; Dénes, A.; Dogan, Y.; Hajdari, A.; Kalle, R.; Reade, B.; Mustafa, B.; Nedelcheva, A.; et al. An ethnobotanical perspective on traditional fermented plant foods and beverages in Eastern Europe. *J. Ethnopharmacol.* **2015**, *170*, 284–296. [CrossRef]
93. Wouters, D.; Grosu-Tudor, S.; Zamfir, M.; De Vuyst, L. Bacterial community dynamics, lactic acid bacteria species diversity and metabolite kinetics of traditional Romanian vegetable fermentations. *J. Sci. Food Agric.* **2013**, *93*, 749–760. [CrossRef]
94. Padonou, W.S.; Nielsen, D.S.; Hounhouigan, J.D.; Thorsen, L.; Nago, M.C.; Jakobsen, M. The microbiota of Lafun, an African traditional cassava food product. *Int. J. Food Microbiol.* **2009**, *133*, 22–30. [CrossRef]
95. Peng, Q.; Jiang, S.; Chen, J.; Ma, C.; Huo, D.; Shao, Y.; Zhang, J. Unique Microbial Diversity and Metabolic Pathway Features of Fermented Vegetables from Hainan, China. *Front. Microbiol.* **2018**, *9*, 399. [CrossRef] [PubMed]
96. Wuyts, S.; Van Beeck, W.; Oerlemans, E.F.M.; Wittouck, S.; Claes, I.J.J.; De Boeck, I.; Weckx, S.; Lievens, B.; De Vuyst, L.; Lebeer, S. Carrot juice fermentations as man-made microbial ecosystems dominated by lactic acid bacteria. *Appl. Environ. Microbiol.* **2018**, *84*. [CrossRef] [PubMed]
97. Beganović, J.; Kos, B.; Leboš Pavunc, A.; Uroić, K.; Jokić, M.; Šušković, J. Traditionally produced sauerkraut as source of autochthonous functional starter cultures. *Microbiol. Res.* **2013**. [CrossRef] [PubMed]
98. Di Cagno, R.; Surico, R.F.; Paradiso, A.; De Angelis, M.; Salmon, J.-C.; Buchin, S.; De Gara, L.; Gobbetti, M. Effect of autochthonous lactic acid bacteria starters on health-promoting and sensory properties of tomato juices. *Int. J. Food Microbiol.* **2009**, *128*, 473–483. [CrossRef] [PubMed]
99. Fessard, A.; Bourdon, E.; Payet, B.; Remize, F. Identification, stress tolerance, and antioxidant activity of lactic acid bacteria isolated from tropically grown fruits and leaves. *Can. J. Microbiol.* **2016**, *62*, 550–561. [CrossRef]
100. Capozzi, V.; Fragasso, M.; Romaniello, R.; Berbegal, C.; Russo, P.; Spano, G.; Capozzi, V.; Fragasso, M.; Romaniello, R.; Berbegal, C.; et al. Spontaneous food fermentations and potential risks for human health. *Fermentation* **2017**, *3*, 49. [CrossRef]

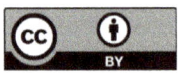

© 2019 by the authors. Licensee MDPI, Basel, Switzerland. This article is an open access article distributed under the terms and conditions of the Creative Commons Attribution (CC BY) license (http://creativecommons.org/licenses/by/4.0/).

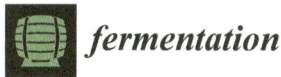

Review

Discovering the Health Promoting Potential of Fermented Papaya Preparation—Its Future Perspectives for the Dietary Management of Oxidative Stress During Diabetes

Jhoti Somanah [1], Manish Putteeraj [1], Okezie I. Aruoma [2,3] and Theeshan Bahorun [4,*]

1. School of Health Sciences, University of Technology, Mauritius, La Tour Koenig, Pointe aux Sables 11134, Mauritius; mjbhugowandeen@umail.utm.ac.mu (J.S.); mputteeraj@umail.utm.ac.mu (M.P.)
2. Department of Undergraduate Studies, College of Science and Integrated Health, Southern California University of Health Sciences, Whittier, CA 90604, USA; oaruoma@calstatela.edu
3. Department of Chemistry and Biochemistry, California State University Los Angeles, Los Angeles, CA 90032, USA
4. ANDI Center of Excellence for Biomedical and Biomaterials Research, University of Mauritius, Réduit 80835, Mauritius
* Correspondence: tbahorun@uom.ac.mu; Tel.: +230-4675-582

Received: 24 July 2018; Accepted: 27 September 2018; Published: 28 September 2018

Abstract: The simplistic morphological characteristics of *Carica papaya* fruit or "pawpaw" should not be the cause for underestimating its potential as a nutraceutical. The market for papaya has been expanding at a staggering rate, partly due to its applicability as a biofortified product, but also due to its phytochemical properties and traditional health benefits. Papaya or formulations of fermented papaya promotion (FPP) display effective free radical scavenging abilities thought to be influenced by its phenolic, carotenoid, flavonoid, or amino acid profile. The antioxidant properties of FPP have been extensively reported in literature to potently target a broad spectrum of free radical-induced diseases ranging from neurological impairments, such as senile dementia, to systemic diseases, to its interference at the cellular level and the support of normal biological ageing processes. FPP has thus been extensively investigated for its ability to exert cellular protective effects and reduce oxidative stress via the mitigation of genetic damage, reduction of lipid peroxidation, and enzymatic inactivation in specific diseases. The focus of this review is to appraise the potential of oxidative stress reduction strategies of FPP and discuss its holistic approach in disease prevention and management, with a particular focus on diabetes and cancer. However, with the current lack of information surrounding its mechanism of action, this review wishes to set the stage and aspire researchers to more profoundly investigate molecular pathways related to how FPP can unequivocally contribute to wellness in an aging population.

Keywords: *Carica papaya*; fermented papaya preparation (FPP); free radical scavenging; antioxidant; oxidative stress; anti-diabetic; anti-carcinogenic

1. Introduction

Being favored for their unique flavor, texture, or health-promoting benefits, fermented foods can be prepared and consumed in a number of ways. One of the important outcomes of food fermentation is its enrichment with essential amino acids, vitamins, and minerals; for example, idli (an Indian cake made from *Rhizopus oligosporous* fermented rice and black-gram) contains high levels of thiamine and riboflavin [1]. Similarly, natto (a sticky soybean dish) is popular amongst the Japanese for its vitamin K2 [2], as is the Nepalese dish of Gundruk (fermented mustard, radish, and cauliflower leaves), which has a high ascorbic acid and fiber content, and *tempeh*, a popular fermented food in Indonesia that is rich in nutrients and active substances [3], with both having a continued consumer appeal worldwide. The process of fermentation coaxes microorganisms into degrading anti-nutritive compounds, making food more edible and digestible, thus augmenting the bioavailability of its health-protecting nutrients. Detoxification, on the other hand, is a sub-process of fermentation, which can render certain foods safer to eat, for example, in the case of cyanogenic glucoside removal from the cassava root by *Geotricum candida* and *Cornibacterium lactii* cultures [4].

Fermented papaya preparation (FPP) is a proprietary yeast fermentation product sold under the commercial trade name of Immun'Âge®. FPP is a certified natural health product and has gained global recognition following its manufacture under the strictest food safety management systems (FSSC 22000 & ISO standards) [5]. Fresh ripe fruit pulp of Hawaiian-grown *Carica papaya* is used for the fabrication of FPP, which is allowed to ferment in the presence of food-grade yeast for up to 12 months. The final product is granulated before being packaged and distributed. Although the general composition of FPP has been ascertained by the Japan Food Research Laboratory, recognition of the presence of several amino acids and novel uncharacterized oligosaccharides in FPP is suspected to be an outcome of the prolonged fermentation process [5]. Studies scrutinizing the therapeutic qualities of papaya fruit have accredited them to its remarkable free radical scavenging activity. At the same time, to explain the source of papaya's antioxidant activity, some authors correlate the latter to its polyphenolic content. Initial fractionation of FPP by Rimbach et al. [6] brought to light the different activity patterns of high- and low-molecular weight fractions with respect to superoxide anion scavenging and macrophage RAW 264.7 activation. Interestingly, Fibach and Ginsburg [7] pointed out that although the overall quantity of phenols in FPP is very low when measured in a salt solution, its levels can be boosted six-fold when assayed in saliva, albumin, mucin, or red blood cell suspensions in vivo. Chemical analysis by Japanese researchers on a fermented papaya preparation using capillary electrophoresis-time-of-flight mass spectrometry (CE-TOFMS) and liquid chromatography (LC-TOFMS) revealed the presence of several low-molecular weight phenolic acids, such as 2,5 dihydroxybenzoic acid, quinic acid, shikimic acid, and m-aminophenol [8]. Although the work of Fujita et al. [5] is amongst the few to shed light on the composition of a fermented papaya preparation, caution must be sought when comparing its outcomes to that of FPP. Disparity in terms of polyphenolic composition and bioactivity will vary as an obvious result of genetic differences between papaya species, cultivation practices, microclimates, and fermentation protocol [8–11]. Furthermore, despite controversy over the sophistication of present analytical technologies and the unelucidated components responsible for the activity of FPP, the authors are in agreement that the multifunctional properties of FPP cannot be singled out to a specific chemical, but rather to a synergistic interaction of its ingredients, which renders it a unique fermented functional food.

2. The Concept of Oxidative Stress as a Unique Therapeutic Pathway by Nutraceuticals for the Management of Type 2 Diabetes

Profound interest in the relationship between free radicals and oxidative stress in diabetes is an area attracting much attention from scientists. During type 2 diabetes, oxidative stress can emerge from the production of free radicals as a result of glucose auto-oxidation, protein glycosylation, low-grade inflammation, and from the metabolic breakdown of free fatty acids [12]. Although the quantity of free radicals generated through normal cellular metabolism is minute, they play a vital regulatory role in many biological processes [13,14]. Environmental factors such as air contaminants, exposure to heavy metals and pesticides, vigorous exercise, and infections are also potential sources of free radicals within the body [15]. Hyperglycemia-induced oxidative stress is believed to be closely associated with the impairment of antioxidant defense mechanisms, representing a central contribution to the onset, progression, and pathology of diabetes and its associated health complications. Defective insulin signaling pathways, degranulation, and accelerated apoptosis of pancreatic β-cells are tell-tale signs of severe oxidative stress in hyperglycemia states [16–18]. Strict weight loss and exercise regimes have been proved to be highly efficient in improving β-cell function, insulin sensitivity, and skeletal muscle oxidative capacity—emphasizing the necessity of maintaining body mass within acceptable levels [19,20]. However, with current sedentary lifestyles, this is an attitude that is unfortunately easier said than done.

Oxidative stress can rapidly overwhelm the activity of endogenous antioxidant enzymes, leaving the body prone to free radical attack, hence the implication of reactive oxygen species in the pathogenesis of several complications associated with diabetes, including heart disease, nephropathy, and retinopathy, is now widely accepted [21–23]. Conjointly, oxidative damage to the structure of DNA can impinge spontaneous mutations, trigger abnormal cell growth, or force premature cell death, provoking the onset of accelerated premature aging and cancer [24]. The common belief that oxidative stress can critically weaken the antioxidant defense system of diabetics has been the center of focus amongst the medical community. The healthful role of natural dietary antioxidants has been discredited in the past, but accumulating evidence obtained from both animal and human experimental models has clearly demonstrated their efficacy to counteract the deleterious effects of oxidative stress in major organs. Compared to conventional anti-diabetes drug therapies, many locally-grown phytonutraceuticals that possess eminent antioxidant powers and exert minimum toxicity are relatively cheap to process, thus offering economically feasible treatment options that can be made accessible worldwide. FPP is one such health product that has gained some criticism, despite overwhelming evidence to support its potential to be an adjunct for the dietary management of oxidative stress in many disease states, as will be highlighted further in this review.

2.1. Interaction of FPP at the Physiological and Organ System Levels in Diabetes

Although an increasing number of plants are being scientifically documented for their anti-hyperglycemic, antioxidant, and insulin stimulating activities [25], scientific evidence supporting the anti-diabetic properties of *Carica papaya* is now accumulating. The anti-hyperglycemic effect of papaya is thought to target pancreatic β cells by improving their sensitivity to insulin, at the same time inhibiting α-amylase and α-glucosidase, a response which bears much resemblance to a second-generation sulfonylurea called glibenclamide [26]. Indeed, there exist many anti-hyperglycemic drugs that normalize plasma glucose levels, but there is a dearth of drugs that show the simultaneous correction of blood glucose, lipid, and antioxidant profiles. Interest in the investigation of the hypoglycemic properties of FPP in diabetic patients was initially investigated by Danese et al. [27] in an open randomized clinical trial in which 3 g FPP/day/2 months was reported to significantly reduce fasting and post-meal glucose levels in both normal and type 2 diabetic patients. These findings were further supported by Collard and Roy [28], where FPP (0.2 g/kg BW/8 weeks) was also found to attenuate the gain in blood glucose in db/db mice. Although these findings do not directly prove the anti-diabetes activity of FPP, they are nonetheless consistent with the hypothesis that FPP can be administrated as an adjuvant treatment option to work in synergy with oral hypoglycemic drugs. While most diabetes-related clinical trials focus on single-target drugs, only a small percent of them are concerned with diabetes prevention, screening, or health maintenance [29]. Diabetes care organizations such as the International Diabetes Federation and American Diabetes Association continuously argue that researchers should prioritize finding more innovative preventive strategies that can work safely in conjunction with conventional diabetes therapies to improve their bioefficacy. In this context, a randomized clinical trial was conducted by our team to accelerate the translation of findings obtained from antioxidant assays conducted on fermented papaya preparation [30–32]. The results of our clinical study demonstrated that a daily supplementation of FPP for three months could improve the general total antioxidant status of pre-diabetic adults (Figure 1) and reduce carbonyl protein levels in plasma [31,33] (Figure 2). In addition, changes in liver biomarkers AST and ALT were also observed [33]. This trend was along the line of findings reported by Santiago et al. [34], who also saw the normalization of ALT and AST by FPP consumption. Elevated enzymes such as ALT, and to a lesser extent AST, can provide insight into the pathology of the liver since it is one of the most susceptible organs to oxidative-related cellular damage, thus helping to predict the risk of developing type 2 diabetes or non-alcoholic fatty liver disease—both of which are on the rise amongst adults within the age range tested [35]. As with all in-vivo studies, a note of caution is required when extrapolating data from clinical studies as drawbacks such as short observation periods, small sample sizes, compliance issues, and differences in analytical techniques need to be considered whilst interpreting findings. However, despite this, it is recommended that medical organizations integrate a variety of such biomarkers into their routine screening exercise protocols for better identification and tracking of at-risk individuals.

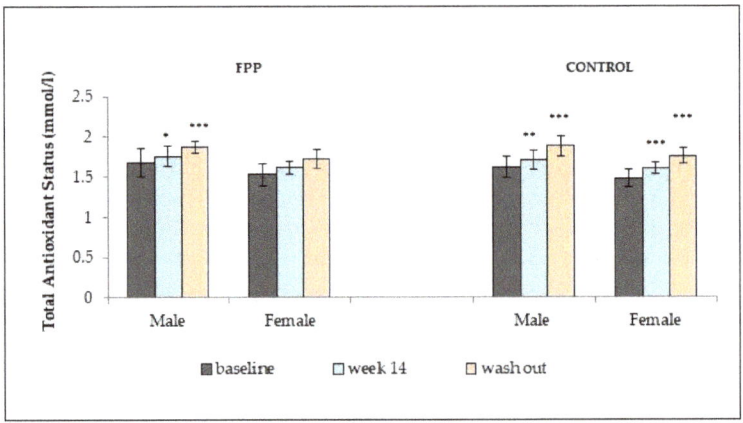

Figure 1. Effect of the total antioxidant (TAS) status in a pre-diabetic population under the FPP ($N = 36$) and control regimes ($N = 53$). Data is expressed as mean TAS value (mmol/L), where error bars represent standard deviation. * $p < 0.05$, ** $p < 0.01$, *** $p < 0.001$ vs. baseline. Reproduced with permission from Somanah et al. [33], Journal of Preventive Medicine; published by Elsevier, 2012.

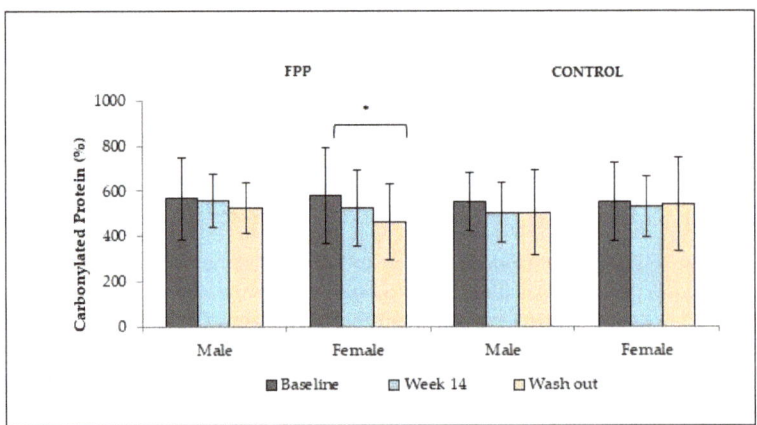

Figure 2. The effect of fermented papaya preparation (FPP) on carbonyl protein accumulation as a percentage compared to control (1% NaCl) in a pre-diabetic population under the FPP ($N = 41$) and control regimes ($N = 58$); error bars represent standard deviation. * $p < 0.05$ vs. baseline. Reproduced with permission from Somanah et al. [31], Food and Chemical Toxicology; published by Elsevier, 2014.

2.2. Anti-Inflammatory and Immuno-Modulatory Effects of FPP in Diabetic Conditions

An observational study published in the American Journal of Human Genetics by Holmes et al. [36] claimed that "for every 1 kg/m² gain in body mass index (BMI), the risk of developing type 2 diabetes increases by 27%"—supporting the notion that type 2 diabetes is a direct outcome of high BMI and increased abdominal fat mass—two major characteristics of obesity which have been linked to sub-clinical inflammatory states in the adipose tissue [37]. In an attempt to understand the influence of oxidative stress on the metabolic response of adipocytes in the presence of papaya, our team used an in vitro cellular model to mimic the micro-environment of metabolic overload by mitochondrial oxidative stress. Using an extract of Mauritian *Carica papaya* (var. Solo), fruit extracts were found to significantly reduce oxidative stress levels within human pre-adipocytes (SW-872). The maintenance of mitochondrial viability, reduction of intracellular reactive oxygen species levels, and mediation of pro-inflammatory cytokine secretory levels (TNF-a, IL-6, MCP-1) were confirmation of papaya's diverse cytoprotective effects against oxidative-inflammation [38]. Similar trends have also been reported in literature for FPP. Papain isolated from the latex of unripe papaya pulp is documented for its anti-bacterial and fibrinolytic properties and used in wound care and chronic skin ulcer therapy for diabetics [39]. In a study by Collard and Roy [28], the authors found that FPP could also accelerate wound healing in db/db mice through its elevation of nitric oxide levels, IL-6, TNF-α, and circulating CD38 at the wound site. Moreover, unexpected surges in TNF-α within SW-872 cells and RAW 269.7 macrophages have been noted by Somanah et al. [38] and Rimbach et al. [6] under immunocompromised states, which were consequently attenuated by FPP. Taken together, these findings suggest that FPP does have unique immunoregulatory effects that can be indicative of its immune system enhancement properties. The gap of knowledge in this area warrants the imperative need to understand its mechanism of action at the molecular level in order for us to support its clinical efficacy claims.

3. Attenuating Type 2 Diabetes Associated Diseases Using the Anti-Oxidant Properties of FPP

At the genomic level, the interaction between oxidative stress mechanisms and chronic inflammation is highly complex, but they are agreed to play pivotal roles in the pathophysiology of diabetes [40]. Therapeutic interventions involving antioxidants could theoretically reduce the risks of base mutations and vulnerability of cells to undergo cell transformation, and lower the susceptibility of erythrocytes to undergo hemolysis reduced during diabetes. The ability of FPP to counteract oxidative stress in human erythrocytes was proven in a randomized supplementation study, where a dose of 6 g FPP/day for a period of 14 weeks clinically reduced the rate of haemolysis and accumulation of protein carbonyls (in-vivo indices of oxidative stress) in the blood plasma of pre-diabetic adults [31] (Figure 2). This finding compliments that reported in Raffaelli et al. [41], where FPP improved platelet function, by enhancing Na^+/K^+-ATPase activity and membrane fluidity, and ameliorated the antioxidant system functionality, through an increase in total antioxidant capacity and SOD activity, and a parallel decrease in conjugated diene levels in patients with type 2 diabetes. Moreover, through a multitude of in-vitro assays, our group has also demonstrated that FPP exhibits potent free radical scavenging potentials that are consistent with those ascribed to FPP in literature [31]. Such positive outcomes strongly suggest FPP to be a therapeutic functional food that can improve the integrity and quality of blood products in pre-diabetics and diabetics.

Taking the electron spin resonance data of Aruoma et al. [42] and Yoshino et al. [43] into consideration, the antioxidant activity of FPP was originally ascribed to its hydroxyl scavenging and iron chelating properties, but this theory has been further extended to its modulatory effects of mitogen-activated protein kinases (MAPKs) and the modification of key antioxidant enzymes such as glutathione peroxidase, SOD, 8-oxoguanine glycosylase, and heme oxygenase 1, amongst others [42,44], and also its polyphenols. Polyphenols have been heavily investigated for their roles in glucose metabolism and buffering against insulin resistance features. Nieto Calvache et al. [45] showed a mixture of soluble and insoluble dietary fibers along with carotenoids, ascorbic acid, and phenolic compounds to be present in papaya, providing evidential support to the characterization of FPP, as reported by [30]. Furthermore, the intestinal bioavailability of these polyphenols in a dietary fibre concentrate was capped to have 65% similarity to the pharmacokinetic properties of the diabetic drug metformin [46]. On a broader scale, components of the *Carica papaya* have been found to decrease serum glucose, triglycerides, and transaminases in STX-induced diabetic rats [47] and positively influence vascular functions and reduce insulin resistance in human subjects [48]. Studies by Martini et al. [49] have shown the ability of polyphenols in upregulating the transcriptional activity of paraoxonase I (PON1), potentially via its protective effects against oxidative stress-induced inactivation, hence altering the pathophysiological processes of diabetes. Other intricate mechanisms have associated polyphenols with improved insulin sensitivity via AMPK activation and the modulation of energy sensors [50]; downregulation of *mIRNA-335* expression to improve insulin signaling and lipid metabolism via the disinhibition of genes such as *InsR, Irs1, Sirt1, Prkaa1, Ppargc1a, Ppara, Lpl, Foxo1*, and *Gsk3b* [51].

FPP exhibits enormous potential towards a more holistic approach in the treatment of diabetes-associated diseases. Combination therapy using metformin and ascorbic acid has been effective in the reduction of depressive behaviors by decreasing corticosterone levels via AMPK pathways in the hypothalamic-pituitary-adrenal axis and inducing a decrease in pro-inflammatory cytokines such as TNF-α and IL-6, which are also linked to neurological disorders and endothelial dysfunction [52].

Oral Health Challenges Amongst the Diabetic Community: Examining the Anti-Cariogenic Potential of FPP

The occurrence of dental caries amongst diabetics is a major health concern, especially when considering the high costs involved in the treatment and management of oral health. Consensus from epidemiological reports is that there has been a sharp increase in the prevalence of oral health complications amongst type 2 diabetics, particularly cases of dental caries, periodontitis, and halitosis [53]. Given the frequency at which these disorders occur amongst the diabetic population, they are now recognized to be part of a multitude of secondary complications manifested during uncontrolled diabetes. The histopathological evidence of the influence of high blood glucose levels on dental caries formation gathered from studies using animal models of diabetes such as alloxan-induced F344 rats [54], WBN/KObSIC rats [55], and db/db mice [56] is evidence of this. Based on the work of Campbell et al. [57], which demonstrated the different types of sugars present in the saliva of diabetics, included lactose, sucrose, fructose, maltose, sorbose, arabinose, and galacturonic acid. It is understood that many of these sugars will remain unnaturally high in the blood of those suffering from uncontrolled diabetes, making the elimination of biofilms difficult [58]. This could explain why diabetics are more susceptible to oral caries, bad breath, and reoccurring mouth infections compared to non-diabetics (Figure 3). Hence, in quest for innovative methods to maintain good oral health of diabetics, researchers have integrated plant extracts into toothpaste, mouthwash, and chewing gum formulations. The use of natural plant-based products for the dietary control and prevention of tooth decay is now favored [59]. However, despite numerous in-vitro studies, only a handful of plants reach clinical testing phases due to their limited effectiveness, stability, taste, and economic feasibility.

Based on Figure 3, recognition of the positive correlation between high levels of blood glucose, inflammatory responses, and the progression of dental caries allows us to theoretically assume that a reduction of key microorganisms in the dental biofilm community is a step towards the reestablishment of oral health in diabetics. This theory was the basis of a study by our group where FPP was examined for its anti-caries properties [30]. Using in vitro simulation models of dental plaque bacterial growth and the hydrophobicity of three opportunistic bacteria, namely *S. mutans, S. mitis*, and *L. acidophilus*, these bacteria were observed to decrease upon exposure to FPP, suggesting that low doses of this dietary health product may be a suitable candidate to complement good oral hygiene practices [30]. The fine powdery consistency of FPP in combination with its high dissolvability not only facilitates its consumption, but also stimulates the secretion of copious quantities of saliva in the mouth. Walsh et al. [60] claim that saliva has a buffering effect on oral biofilms. The secretion of copious amounts of saliva in the mouth by FPP would therefore imply the rapid clearance of large food debris and encourage the buccal pH to return to the baseline. In a study by Fibach and Ginsburg, the authors pointed out that an individual's oxidative stress level has an influential role to play in the health status of their oral cavity. Employing two highly sensitive luminol-dependent chemiluminescence assays, the authors demonstrated that under pathological conditions, FPP could easily dissolve in saliva or red blood cells to augment their antioxidant capacities [7]. The study conducted by our group and reported in Somanah et al. [33] clearly supports this theory, and hence FPP may have a role in oral health benefits. Interestingly, one previous study has reported that the consumption of FPP indeed led to an increased rate of salivary secretions high in IgA and phase II enzymes [61]. With regards to periodontitis in diabetics (a chronic bucal infection largely caused by the pathogen *Porphyromonas gingivalis*), the detection of abnormal levels of TNF-α, IL-6, IL-1β, and CRP in gingival fluid and tissue indicates that this condition is characterized by chronic inflammation which is hypothesized to lead to the progressive destruction of the tissues supporting the teeth, cementum, and alveolar bone. In a recent open randomized study, Russian investigators proved the clinical efficacy of a fermented papaya gel against periodontitis. Topical administration of this gel was observed to lead to a considerable improvement of major indices of disease severity, such as reduced bleeding and gingival pocket depth, and the normalization of IL-10, IL-6, and IL-1β cytokine levels after 14 days of application, all of which may be of direct relevance to diabetics (Figure 3). Although the exact mechanism has yet to be understood, the authors speculate that FPP can work in synergy with human granulocytes to enhance the phagocytosis of key microorganisms present in gingival tissues [62].

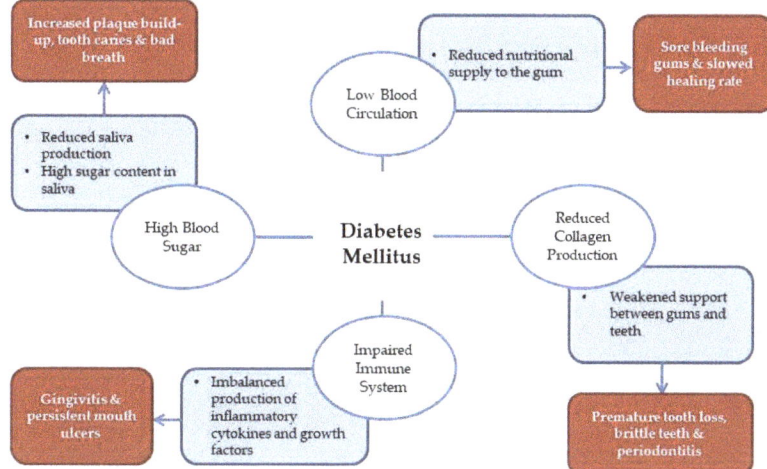

Figure 3. Common reasons as to why diabetics are prone to developing oral health issues.

Unfortunately, the lack of studies investigating the anti-cariogenic potential of FPP renders a comparative discussion of its possible mechanisms of action difficult. Attention has instead been given to papain-containing formulations from fresh fruit extracts [63] as their nutritional and biochemical composition is thought to be less complex than that of FPP. The anti-cariogenic activity of papain has been observed to be highly selective, only acting upon carious tissue, which does not express genes encoding for a plasmatic protease inhibitor: alpha 1 anti-trypsin [63]. Whether this characteristic can be observed by FPP remains to be explored. Nevertheless, papaya-based products show a promising perspective for future studies in the area of phytodentistry.

4. Appreciating the Anti-Cancer Effects Precipitated by FPP

Despite large investments made in the area of cancer prevention, the escalating prevalence of cancer amongst diabetics clearly indicates that the present success rate of clinical therapies is low. One prominent explanation for this is that preclinical research on anti-cancer drugs is flawed, in the sense that it overlooks treating the fundamental cause of cancer: oxidative stress. Recognition between prolonged oxidative-inflammatory insults during diabetes as the etiology of cancer has sparked our interest in searching for natural but innovative anti-cancer agents. Understanding how the diabetes micro-environment can predispose one to the onset of cancer has been reviewed by our group in Aruoma et al. [64], bringing forward the concept that ROS- and cytokine-dependent signaling pathways represent a specific vulnerability that can be selectively targeted by antioxidants. Novel bioactive components such as benzyl glucosinolate, which exhibit anti-growth activities on several tumor cell lines, have been identified in papaya [65]. The review paper of Nguyen et al. [66] explores the anticancer activities attributed to organic extracts of papaya.

In light of the previous sections which lengthily discuss the pertinence of FPP to modulate biomarkers of oxidative stress and inflammation within cell-based models, the eventual goal of our group was to shed light on the anti-cancer propensity of the papaya-based product—FPP. Common combinational therapies include surgery, chemotherapy, radiation, and immunosuppressant drugs, which are deemed effective, but highly aggressive. Unpleasant side-effects such as acute headaches, vomiting, nausea, and occasional bouts of unconsciousness are commonly experienced by patients. Also, with exposure to high levels of ionizing radiation, severe oxidative stress can increase the patient's risk to structural damage of the skin, spermatogia, and hematopoietic stem cells, amongst others [67–69]. A group of Russian researchers was amongst the first to notice a positive effect upon the regular consumption of FPP in children undergoing radiotherapy [70], notably in terms of the attenuation of unpleasant side effects associated with aggressive radiotherapy. Referring to published findings of our group in the Journal Life Sciences, the seminal research work of Somanah et al. used the N-methyl-N-nitrosourea (MNU)-injected balb/c mice model to explore the modulatory effect of FPP against MNU-induced hepatocellular carcinoma [71]. Amongst all doses tested, mice of the 500 mg FPP/kg BW group were found to benefit the most from this treatment. Reduced shedding of hair, improved alertness, and a gain in both weight and appetite were noted. Moreover, from a haematological point-of-view, compared to the control group, a subsequent drop of nearly 31% in the haemoglobin level was noted, undoubtedly caused by excessive free radical attack on vulnerable erythrocytes and phase II detoxifying/antioxidant enzymes. Fractions of whole blood such as hemoglobin concentrations, and leukocyte and platelet counts were found to normalize. This is a possible indication of the counter-occurrence of MNU-induced hemolysis by FPP. Furthermore, the platelet count in MNU control mice remained exceptionally high, which was indicative of the formation of metastatic lesions within the liver. This was visually confirmed by the appearance of red, swollen, and inflamed growths on the abdominal area of treated mice. In this study [71], circulating malondialdehyde (MDA) levels (a toxic product of lipid peroxidation which is considered to be indirect tumor promoter and co-carcinogenic agent) were observed to drop (Figure 4), together with simultaneous augmentations in enzymatic SOD (+20%), CAT (+81%), and GPx (+66%) release in FPP-supplemented mice. These findings coincide with similar trends reported previously [44,70,72].

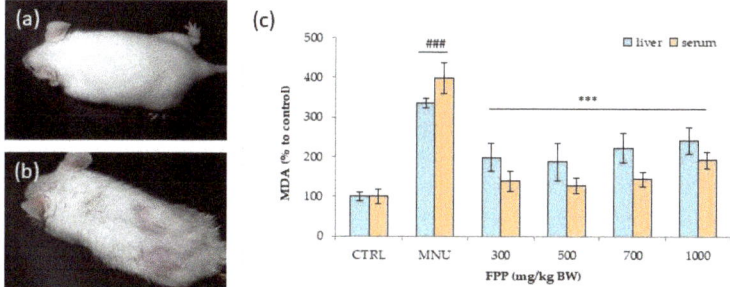

Figure 4. (a) Physical appearance of balb/c mice from the PBS control group and (b) N-methyl-N-nitrosourea (MNU) control group. (c) Malondialdehyde (MDA) levels in fermented papaya preparation (FPP)-supplemented balb/c mice treated with or without MNU. Data is presented as the mean of five replicates, where error bars represent ± standard deviation. ### $p < 0.001$ vs. PBS control; *** $p < 0.001$ vs. MNU control. Reproduced with permission from Somanah et al. [71], Life Sciences; published by Elsevier, 2016.

Although no profound molecular studies have been conducted on FPP to explain how it achieves these outcomes, some theories have been put forward through the use of genotoxins like MNU, benzo(a)pyrene, Fe-NTA, and H_2O_2, which are documented to attack DNA and distort its stability through two basic pathways: either by reaction with a DNA nucleophile or electrophile, or by reaction with the pi (π) or C-H bonds located within nucleotides. This is evidenced by increased peak intensities at 1190, 1254, 1322, 1405, 1152, and 1463 cm^{-1} using Raman laser spectroscopy (Figure 5) [73]. In a unique study, our group utilized Raman laser spectroscopy for the first time to detect any reversal of structural alterations (damage) inflicted by MNU on DNA by FPP. Data showed the reduction in the intensity of peaks at regions corresponding to nucleotide bases or to the phosphodiester backbone (Figure 5) [71]. This provides sufficient evidence that FPP can indeed protect DNA through radical scavenging, as proposed in an earlier study by Aruoma et al. [5] and Rimbach et al. [6]. Molecular data suggests that FPP reduces the extent of DNA damage by enhancing the activation of ERK, p35, and Akt. Such protein kinases are activated in response to DNA damage, providing a cellular signal to DNA repair enzymes (e.g., hOGG1), survival proteins (e.g., bcl-2), cell cycle control factors (e.g., cyclin D1), and several transcription factors [5,44]. FPP is also thought to divert hydroxyl radicals away from the π bonds of C5-C6 pyrimidines and N8-N7 or C4-C8 bonds of purines—thus protecting the vulnerable areas of DNA from any major structural alterations [43,74].

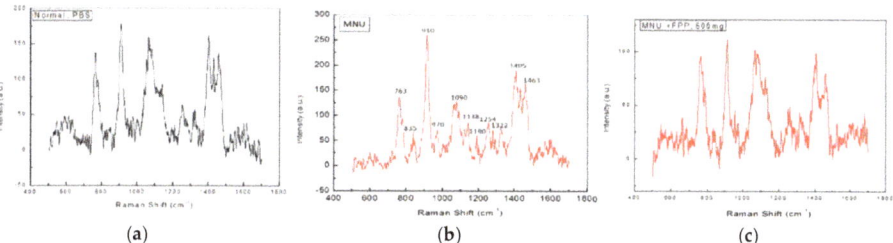

Figure 5. Comparison of Raman laser spectra of liver DNA in the region of 400–1700 cm^{-1} for all experimental groups: (a) PBS control, (b) MNU control, (c) MNU + 500 mg FPP/kg BW. Data is representative of eight replicates. [Parameters: resolution cm^{-1}, step of 100 nm, laser power 5 mW, exciting source 514.5 nm argon ion laser]. Reproduced with permission from Somanah et al. [71], Life Sciences; published by Elsevier, 2016.

The results of the study reported in Somanah et al. [71] clearly suggest that FPP can simultaneously boost the recovery of the immune defense system, hinder DNA damage, and reduce symptoms of ill health associated with aggressive carcinoma. The increased longevity of our test model mice undoubtedly proves that liver cancer can be managed to some extent without any harsh medical intervention. To date, the hepatoprotective effects of FPP have not been explored using this animal model with MNU as a tumorigen. These findings are therefore of great importance to the field of phytochemotherapy. Furthermore, no adverse effects have been noted in the literature to date regarding the consumption of FPP—deeming it safe for both adults and children. Extrapolation of the observations discussed in this paper and those reported by our group thus appraise fermented papaya preparation to be a remarkable yet feasible phytonutraceutical which can be used to prevent or manage diseases governed by chronic oxidative stress, especially diabetes and cancer.

5. Conclusions

Discussions included within this review converge to the bottom line that free radicals do indeed contribute to the surge in chronic diseases in individuals who are burdened by uncontrolled oxidative stress. Studies on FPP have been overlooked by some researchers, as several findings appear inconclusive due to the lack of supplementary evidence of its composition. Nonetheless, the expansive evidence gathered over the past decade presents FPP as an intriguing yet promising health supplement that deserves greater attention from the scientific community. Efforts now need to be steered towards the elucidation of its composition and its mechanistic approach in the diseased micro-environment in order to appreciate its true potential.

Author Contributions: J.S., M.P., O.I.A., and T.B. wrote/reviewed/edited the manuscript.

Funding: The Authors acknowledge the financial support from the Mauritius Research Council under the National Research and Innovation Chair program of T.B.

Conflicts of Interest: O.I.A. is actively involved in biomedical research involving fermented papaya preparation for the Osato Research Institute, Gifu, Japan.

References

1. Ghosh, D.; Chattopadhyay, P. Preparation of idli batter, its properties and nutritional improvement during fermentation. *J. Food Sci. Technol.* **2011**, *48*, 610–615. [CrossRef] [PubMed]
2. Tsukamoto, Y.; Ichise, H.; Kakuda, H.; Yamaguchi, M. Intake of fermented soybean (natto) increases circulating vitamin K_2 (menaquinone-7) and gamma-carboxylated osteocalcin concentration in normal individuals. *J. Bone Miner. Metab.* **2000**, *18*, 216–222. [CrossRef] [PubMed]
3. Dinesh Babu, P.; Bhakyaraj, R.; Vidhyalakshmi, R. A low-cost nutritious food "Tempeh"—A review. *World J. Diary Food Sci.* **2009**, *4*, 22–27.
4. Montagnac, J.; Davis, C.; Tanumihardjo, S. Processing Techniques to Reduce Toxicity and Anti nutrients of Cassava for Use as a Staple Food. *Compr. Rev. Food Sci. Food Saf.* **2009**, *8*, 17–27. [CrossRef]
5. Aruoma, O.I.; Yuki, H.; Marotta, F.; Mantello, P.; Rachmilewitz, E.A.; Montagnier, L. Applications and bioefficacy of the functional food supplement fermented papaya preparation. *Toxicology* **2010**, *278*, 75–87. [CrossRef] [PubMed]
6. Rimbach, G.; Park, Y.C.; Guo, Q.; Moini, H.; Qureshi, N.; Saliou, C.; Takayama, K.; Virgili, F.; Packer, L. Nitric oxide synthesis and TNF-alpha secretion in RAW 264.7 macrophages: Mode of action of a fermented papaya preparation. *Life Sci.* **2000**, *67*, 679–694. [CrossRef]
7. Fibach, E.; Ginsburg, I. The Antioxidant Effect of Fermented Papaya Preparation in the Oral Cavity. *Phytother. Res.* **2015**, *29*, 1317–1322. [CrossRef] [PubMed]
8. Fujita, Y.; Tsuno, H.; Nakayama, J. Fermented Papaya Preparation Restores Age-Related Reductions in Peripheral Blood Mononuclear Cell Cytolytic Activity in Tube-Fed Patients. *PLoS ONE* **2017**, *12*, e0169240. [CrossRef] [PubMed]
9. Maisarah, A.M.; Asmah, R.; Fauziah, O. Proximate analysis, antioxidant and antiproliferative activities of different parts of Carica papaya. *J. Nutr. Food Sci.* **2014**, *4*, 267.

10. Luximon-Ramma, A.; Bahorun, T.; Crozier, A. Antioxidant actions and phenolic and vitamin C contents of common Mauritian exotic fruits. *J. Sci. Food Agric.* **2003**, *83*, 496–502. [CrossRef]
11. Simirgiotis, M.J.; Caligari, P.D.S.; Schmeda-Hirschmann, G. Identification of phenolic compounds from the fruits of the mountain papaya Vasconcellea pubescens A. DC. grown in Chile by liquid chromatography–UV detection–mass spectrometry. *Food Chem.* **2009**, *115*, 775–784. [CrossRef]
12. Moussa, S.A. Oxidative stress in diabetes mellitus. *Rom. J. Biophys.* **2008**, *18*, 225–236.
13. Valko, M.; Leibfritz, D.; Moncol, J.; Cronin, M.T.; Mazur, M.; Telser, J. Free radicals and antioxidants in normal physiological functions and human disease. *Int. J. Biochem. Cell Biol.* **2007**, *39*, 44–84. [CrossRef] [PubMed]
14. Dröge, W. Free radicals in the physiological control of cell function. *Arch. Biochem. Biophys.* **2002**, *430*, 37–48. [CrossRef] [PubMed]
15. Bagchi, K.; Puri, S. Free radicals and antioxidants in health and disease. *East Mediterr. Health J.* **1998**, *4*, 350–360.
16. Rains, J.L.; Jain, S.K. Oxidative stress, insulin signaling, and diabetes. *Free Radic. Biol. Med.* **2011**, *50*, 567–575. [CrossRef] [PubMed]
17. Butler, A.E.; Janson, J.; Bonner-Weir, S.; Ritzel, R.; Rizza, R.A.; Butler, P.C. Beta-cell deficit and increased beta-cell apoptosis in humans with type 2 diabetes. *Diabetes* **2010**, *52*, 102–110. [CrossRef]
18. Finegood, D.T.; Mcarthur, M.D.; Kojwang, D.; Thomas, M.J.; Topp, B.G.; Leonard, T.; Buckingham, R.E. Beta-cell mass dynamics in Zucker diabetic fatty rats. Rosiglitazone prevents the rise in net cell death. *Diabetes* **2001**, *50*, 1021–1029. [CrossRef] [PubMed]
19. Solomon, T.P.; Haus, J.M.; Kelly, K.R.; Rocco, M.; Kashyap, S.R.; Kirwan, J.P. Improved pancreatic beta-cell function in type 2 diabetic patients after lifestyle-induced weight loss is related to glucose-dependent insulinotropic polypeptide. *Diabetes Care* **2010**, *33*, 1561–1566. [CrossRef] [PubMed]
20. Hood, M.S.; Little, J.P.; Tarnopolsky, M.A.; Myslik, F.; Gibala, M.J. Low-volume interval training improves muscle oxidative capacity in sedentary adults. *Med. Sci. Sports Exerc.* **2011**, *43*, 1849–1856. [CrossRef] [PubMed]
21. Fowler, M.J. Microvascular and macrovascular complications of diabetes. *Clin. Diabetes* **2008**, *26*, 77–82. [CrossRef]
22. Mshelia, D.S. Role of free radicals in pathogenesis of diabetes nephropathy. *Ann. Afr. Med.* **2004**, *3*, 55–62.
23. Oloffson, E.A.; Marlund, S.L.; Behnoig, A. Enhanced diabetes induced cataract in copper zinc superoxide dismutase-null mice. *Investig. Ophthalmol. Vis. Sci.* **2009**, *50*, 2913–2918. [CrossRef] [PubMed]
24. Aruoma, O.I. Free radicals, oxidative stress, and antioxidants in human health and disease. *J. Am. Oil. Chem. Soc.* **1998**, *75*, 199–212. [CrossRef]
25. Pandeya, K.B.; Tripathi, I.P.; Mishra, M.K.; Dwivedi, N.; Pardhi, Y.; Kamal, A.; Gupta, P.; Dwivedi, N.; Mishra, C. A Critical Review on Traditional Herbal Drugs: An Emerging Alternative Drug for Diabetes. *Int. J. Org. Chem.* **2013**, *3*, 1–22. [CrossRef]
26. Oboh, G.; Olabiyi, A.A.; Akinyemi, A.J.; Ademiluyi, A.O. Inhibition of key enzymes linked to type 2 diabetes and sodium nitroprusside-induced lipid peroxidation in rat pancreas by water-extractable phytochemicals from unripe pawpaw fruit (*Carica papaya*). *J. Basic Clin. Physiol. Pharmacol.* **2013**, *30*, 1–14. [CrossRef] [PubMed]
27. Danese, C.; Espoisto, D.; D'alfonso, V.; Civene, M.; Ambrosino, M.; Colotto, M. Plasma glucose level decreases as a collateral effect of fermented papaya preparation use. *Clin. Ther.* **2006**, *157*, 195–198.
28. Collard, E.; Roy, S. Improved function of diabetic wound site macrophages and accelerated wound closure in response to oral supplementation of a fermented papaya preparation. *Antioxid. Redox. Signal* **2010**, *13*, 599–606. [CrossRef] [PubMed]
29. Lakey, W.C.; Barnard, K.; Batch, B.C.; Chiswel, L.K.; Tasneem, A.; Green, J.B. Are current clinical trials in diabetes addressing important issues in diabetes care? *Diabetologia* **2013**, *56*, 1226–1235. [CrossRef] [PubMed]
30. Somanah, J.; Bourdon, E.; Bahorun, T.; Aruoma, O.I. The inhibitory effect of a fermented papaya preparation on growth, hydrophobicity, and acid production of *Streptococcus mutans, Streptococcus mitis, and Lactobacillus acidophilus*: Its implications in oral health improvement of diabetics. *Food Sci. Nutr.* **2013**, *1*, 416–421. [CrossRef] [PubMed]

31. Somanah, J.; Bourdon, E.; Rondeau, P.; Bahorun, T.; Aruoma, O.I. Relationship between fermented papaya preparation supplementation, erythrocyte integrity and antioxidant status in pre-diabetics. *Food Chem. Toxicol.* **2014**, *65*, 12–17. [CrossRef] [PubMed]
32. Ghoti, H.; Rosenbaum, H.; Fibach, E.; Rachmilewitz, E.A. Decreased hemolysis following administration of antioxidant—fermented papaya preparation (FPP) to a patient with PNH. *Ann. Hematol.* **2010**, *89*, 429–440. [CrossRef] [PubMed]
33. Somanah, J.; Aruoma, O.I.; Gunness, T.K.; Kowelssur, S.; Dambala, V.; Murad, F.; Googoolye, K.; Daus, D.; Indelicato, J.; Bourdon, E.; et al. Effects of a short term supplementation of a fermented papaya preparation on biomarkers of diabetes mellitus in a randomized Mauritian population. *J. Prev. Med.* **2012**, *54*, S90–S97. [CrossRef] [PubMed]
34. Santiago, L.A.; Uno, K.; Kishida, T.; Miyagawa, F.; Osato, J.A.; Mori, A. Effect of Immun'Age on serum components and immunological functions in humans. *Neurosciences* **1994**, *20*, 149–152.
35. Trojak, A. Nonalcoholic Fatty Liver Disease in Patients with Type 2 Diabetes- Gender Differentiation in Determinants. *J. Diabetes Metab.* **2015**, *6*, 476. [CrossRef]
36. Holmes, M.V.; Lange, L.A.; Palmer, T.; Lanktree, M.B.; North, K.E.; Almoguera, B.; Buxbaum, S.; Chandrupatla, H.R.; Elbers, C.C.; GUO, Y.; et al. Causal effects of body mass index on cardiometabolic traits and events: A Mendelian randomization analysis. *Am. J. Hum. Genet.* **2014**, *94*, 198–208. [CrossRef] [PubMed]
37. Oh, D.Y.; Morinaga, H.; Talukdar, S.; Bae, E.J.; Olefsky, J.M. Increased macrophage migration into adipose tissue in obese mice. *Diabetes* **2012**, *61*, 346–354. [CrossRef] [PubMed]
38. Somanah, J.; Bourdon, E.; Bahorun, T. Extracts of Mauritian *Carica papaya* (var. solo) protect SW872 and HepG2 cells against hydrogen peroxide induced oxidative stress. *J. Food Sci. Technol.* **2017**, *54*, 1917–1927. [CrossRef] [PubMed]
39. Blakytny, R.; Jude, E. The molecular biology of chronic wounds and delayed healing in diabetes. *Diabetic Med.* **2006**, *23*, 594–608. [CrossRef] [PubMed]
40. Houstis, N.; Rosen, E.D.; Lander, E.S. Reactive oxygen species have a casual role in multiple forms of insulin resistance. *Nature* **2006**, *440*, 944–948. [CrossRef] [PubMed]
41. Raffaelli, F.; Nanetti, L.; Montecchiani, G.; Borroni, F.; Salvolini, E.; Faloia, E.; Ferretti, G.; Mazzanti, L.; Vignini, A. In vitro effects of fermented papaya (*Carica papaya*, L.) on platelets obtained from patients with type 2 diabetes. *Nutr. Metab. Cardiovasc. Dis.* **2015**, *25*, 224–229. [CrossRef] [PubMed]
42. Aruoma, O.I.; Colognato, R.; Fontana, I.; Gartlon, J.; Migliore, L.; Koike, K.; Coecke, S.; Lamy, E.; Mersch-Sundermann, V.; Laurenz, I.; et al. Molecular effects of a fermented papaya preparation on oxidative damage, MAP kinase activation and modulation of the benzo [a] pyrene mediated genotoxicity. *Biofactors* **2006**, *26*, 147–159. [CrossRef] [PubMed]
43. Yoshino, F.; Lee, M.C.I.; Kobayashi, K.; Hayashi, Y.; Aruoma, O.I. Assessment of the effect of a fermented papaya preparation on oxidative damage in spontaneously hypertensive rat (SHR) brain using electron spin resonance (ESR) imaging and L-band spectroscopy. *J. Funct. Food* **2009**, *1*, 375–380. [CrossRef]
44. Marotta, F.; Koike, K.; Lorenzetti, A.; Jain, S.; Signorelli, P.; Metugriachuk, Y.; Mantello, P.; Locorotondo, N. Regulating redox balance gene expression in healthy individuals by nutraceuticals: A pilot study. *Rejuv. Res.* **2010**, *13*, 175–178. [CrossRef] [PubMed]
45. Calvache, J.; Cueto, M.; Farroni, A.; De Escalada, P.M.; Gerschenson, L.N. Antioxidant characterization of new dietary fiber concentrates from Papaya pulp and peel (*Carica papaya* L.). *J. Funct. Foods* **2016**, *27*, 319–328. [CrossRef]
46. Scheen, A.J. Clinical pharmacokinetics of metformin. *Clin. Pharmacokinet.* **1996**, *30*, 359–371. [CrossRef] [PubMed]
47. Juárez-Rojop, I.E.; Tovilla-Zárate, C.A.; Aguilar-Domínguez, D.E.; Fuente, L.F.; Lobato-García, C.E.; Blé-Castillo, J.L.; López-Meraz, L.; Díaz-Zagoya, J.C.; Bermúdez-Ocaña, D.Y. Phytochemical screening and hypoglycemic activity of *Carica papaya* leaf in streptozotocin-induced diabetic rats. *Rev. Bras. Farmacogn.* **2014**, *24*, 341–347. [CrossRef]
48. Cao, H.; Wang, Y.; Xiao, J. Dietary Polyphenols and Type 2 Diabetes: Human Study and Clinical Trial. *Free Radic. Biol. Med.* **2017**, *112*, 158. [CrossRef]
49. Martini, D.; Del Bo', C.; Porrini, M.; Ciappellano, S.; Riso, P. Role of polyphenols and polyphenol-rich foods in the modulation of PON1 activity and expression. *J. Nutr. Biochem.* **2017**, *48*, 1–8. [CrossRef] [PubMed]

50. Mutlur, K.R.; Carani, V.A. Polyphenols activate energy sensing network in insulin resistant models. *Chem. Biol. Interact.* **2017**, *275*, 95–107. [CrossRef] [PubMed]
51. Otton, R.; Bolin, A.P.; Ferreira, L.T.; Marinovic, M.P.; Rocha, A.L.S.; Mori, M.A. Polyphenol-rich green tea extract improves adipose tissue metabolism by down-regulating miR-335 expression and mitigating insulin resistance and inflammation. *J. Nutr. Biochem.* **2018**, *57*, 170–179. [CrossRef] [PubMed]
52. Shivavedi, N.; Kumar, M.; Tej, G.N.V.C.; Nayak, P.K. Metformin and ascorbic acid combination therapy ameliorates type 2 diabetes mellitus and comorbid depression in rats. *Brain Res.* **2017**, *1674*, 1–9. [CrossRef] [PubMed]
53. Bajaj, S.; Prasad, S.; Gupta, A.; Singh, V.B. Oral manifestations in type 2 diabetes and related complications. *Indian J. Endocrinol. Metab.* **2012**, *16*, 777–779. [CrossRef] [PubMed]
54. Nakahara, Y.; Sano, T.; Kodama, Y.; Ozaki, K.; Matsura, T. Allozan-induced hyoerglycemia causes rapid onset and progressive dental caries and periodontitis in F344 rats. *Histol. Histopathol.* **2012**, *27*, 1297–1306. [PubMed]
55. Kodama, Y.; Matsurura, M.; Sanyo, T.; Nakaraha, Y.; Ozaki, K.; Narama, I.; Matsuura, T. Diabetes enhances dental caries and apical periodontitis in caries susceptible WBN/KobSIc rats. *J. Complement. Med.* **2011**, *61*, 53–59.
56. Sano, T.; Matsuura, T.; Ozaki, K.; Narama, I. Dental caries and caries-related periodontitis in type 2 diabetic mice. *Vet. Pathol.* **2011**, *48*, 506–512. [CrossRef] [PubMed]
57. Campbell, M.J.A. Glucose in the saliva of the non-diabetic and the diabetic patient. *Arch. Oral Biol.* **1965**, *10*, 197–205. [CrossRef]
58. Loë, H. Periodontal disease: The sixth complication of diabetes mellitus. *Diabetes Care* **1993**, *16*, 329–334. [CrossRef] [PubMed]
59. Hotwani, K.; Baliga, S.; Sharma, K. Phytodentistry: Use of medicinal plants. *J. Complement. Integr. Med.* **2014**, *11*, 233–251. [CrossRef] [PubMed]
60. Walsh, L.J. Clinical dental plaque fermentation and its role in caries risk assessment. *Int. J. Dent.* **2006**, *8*, 34–40.
61. Marotta, F.; Naito, Y.; Jain, S.; Lorenzetti, A.; Soresi, V.; Kumari, A.; Carrera Bastos, P.; Tomella, C.; Yadav, H. Is there a potential application of a fermented nutraceutical in acute respiratory illnesses? An in-vivo placebo-controlled, cross-over clinical study in different age groups of healthy subjects. *J. Biol. Regul. Homeost. Agents* **2012**, *26*, 285–294. [PubMed]
62. Kharaeva, Z.F.; Zhanimova, LR.; Mustafaev, M.S.; De Luca, C.; Mayer, W.; Thai, J.C.S.; Tuan, R.T.S.; Korkina, L.G. Effects of Standardised Fermented Papaya Gel on Clinical Symptoms, Inflammatory Cytokines, and Nitric Oxide Metabolites in Patients with Chronic Periodontitis: An Open Randomized Clinical Study. *Mediators Inflamm.* **2016**, *2016*, 9379840. [CrossRef] [PubMed]
63. Bhardwaj, A.; Bhardwaj, S.V. Papacarie® containing papain: A natural chemomechanical caries removal agent. *Res. J. Pharm. Biol. Chem. Sci.* **2012**, *3*, 660–665.
64. Aruoma, O.I.; Neergheen, V.S.; Bahorun, T.; Jen, L.-S. Free Radicals, Antioxidants and Diabetes: Embryopathy, Retinopathy, Neuropathy, Nephropathy and Cardiovascular Complications. *Neuroembryol. Aging* **2006**, *4*, 117–137. [CrossRef]
65. Li, Z.-Y.; Wang, Y.; Shen, W.-T.; Zhou, P. Content determination of benzyl glucosinolate and anti-cancer activity of its hydrolysis product in *Carica papaya* L. *Asian Pac. J. Trop. Dis.* **2012**, *5*, 231–233. [CrossRef]
66. Nguyen, T.T.; Shaw, P.N.; Parat, M.O.; Hewavitharana, A.K. Anticancer activity of Carica Papaya: A Review. *Mol. Nutr. Food Res.* **2013**, *57*, 153–164. [CrossRef] [PubMed]
67. Bickers, D.R.; Athar, M. Oxidative stress in the pathogenesis of skin disease. *J. Investig. Dermatol.* **2006**, *126*, 2565–2575. [CrossRef] [PubMed]
68. Ahmadi, A.; Ng, S.-C. Fertilizing ability of DNA-damaged spermatozoa. *J. Exp. Zool.* **1999**, *284*, 696–704. [CrossRef]
69. Wang, Y.; Liu, L.; Pazhanisamy, S.K.; Li, H.; Meng, A.; Zhou, D. Total body irradiation causes residual bone marrow injury by induction of persistent oxidative stress in murine hematopoietic stem cells. *Free Rad. Biol. Med.* **2010**, *48*, 348–356. [CrossRef] [PubMed]
70. Korkindel, L.; Osato, J.A.; Chivilyema, I.; Samocravyova, E.; Cheremisina, Z.; Afanas'ev, I. Radioproetctive and antioxidant effects of zinc aspartate and fpp in aspartate and fpp in Children with acute myelo-iympholeukemia. *Nutrition* **1995**, *11*, 555–558.

71. Somanah, J.; Ramsaha, S.; Verma, S.; Kumar, A.; Sharma, P.; Singh, R.K.; Aruoma, O.I.; Bourdon, E.; Bahorun, T. Fermented papaya preparation modulates the progression of n-methyl-n-nitrosourea induced hepatocellular carcinoma in Balb/C mice. *Life Sci.* **2016**, *151*, 330–338. [CrossRef] [PubMed]
72. Imao, K.; Wang, H.; Komatsu, M.; Hiramatsu, M. Free radical scavenging activity of fermented papaya preparation and its effect on lipid peroxide level and superoxide dismutase activity in iron-induced epileptic foci of rats. *Biochem. Mol. Biol. Int.* **1998**, *45*, 11–23. [CrossRef] [PubMed]
73. Verma, S.; Bahorun, T.; Singh, R.K.; Aruoma, O.I.; Kumar, A. Effect of aegle marmelos leaf extract on n-methyl n-nitrosourea-induced hepatocarcinogensis in Balb/C Mice. *Pharm. Biol.* **2013**, *51*, 1272–1281. [CrossRef] [PubMed]
74. Wood, C.D.; Thornton, T.M.; Sabio, G.; Davis, R.A.; Rincon, M. Nuclear localization of p38 MAPK in response to DNA damage. *Int. J. Biol. Sci.* **2007**, *5*, 428–437. [CrossRef]

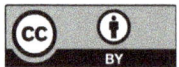

© 2018 by the authors. Licensee MDPI, Basel, Switzerland. This article is an open access article distributed under the terms and conditions of the Creative Commons Attribution (CC BY) license (http://creativecommons.org/licenses/by/4.0/).

MDPI
St. Alban-Anlage 66
4052 Basel
Switzerland
Tel. +41 61 683 77 34
Fax +41 61 302 89 18
www.mdpi.com

Fermentation Editorial Office
E-mail: fermentation@mdpi.com
www.mdpi.com/journal/fermentation

www.ingramcontent.com/pod-product-compliance
Lightning Source LLC
LaVergne TN
LVHW071959080526
838202LV00064B/6786